Dental Reception and Practice Management

Dental Reception and Practice Management

Glenys Bridges
Managing Director
Dental Resource Company

Blackwell
Munksgaard

Blackwell Munksgaard, a Blackwell Publishing Company,
Editorial Offices:
Blackwell Publishing Ltd, 9600 Garsington Road, Oxford OX4 2DQ, UK
  Tel: +44 (0)1865 776868
Blackwell Publishing Professional, 2121 State Avenue, Ames, Iowa 50014-8300, USA
  Tel: +1 515 292 0140
Blackwell Publishing Asia Pty Ltd, 550 Swanston Street, Carlton, Victoria 3053, Australia
  Tel: +61 (0)3 8359 1011

First published 2006 by Blackwell Munksgaard

ISBN-13: 978-14051-3888-8
ISBN-10: 1-4051-3888-2

Library of Congress Cataloging-in-Publication Data

Bridges, Glenys, 1956–
  Dental reception and practice management / Glenys Bridges.
    p. ; cm.
  Includes bibliographical references and index.
  ISBN-13: 978-1-4051-3888-8 (pbk. : alk. paper)
  ISBN-10: 1-4051-3888-2 (pbk. : alk. paper)
  1. Dental offices–Management. 2. Receptionists. I. Title.
  [DNLM: 1. Dental Auxiliaries. 2. Practice Management, Dental–organization &
administration. WU 90 B851d 2006]

RK58.B77 2006
617.6'0068–dc22

                                                                      2006013670

A catalogue record for this title is available from the British Library

Set in 10/12.5pt Palatino
by Graphicraft Limited, Hong Kong

For further information on Blackwell Publishing, visit our website:
www.dentistry.blackwellmunksgaard.com

Contents

About the Author

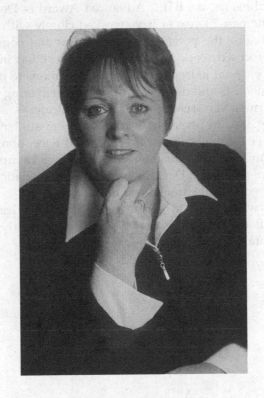

My career in dentistry began in 1972 when as a school leaver I was employed as a dental nurse-receptionist. This was a time when careers in dentistry offered very few prospects or opportunities, unlike the ever-growing range of career prospects for dental care professionals today. My interests lay mostly in the reception work where I could mingle with patients and where the work was more self-determined and less restricted than chairside work.

In 1975, looking for a career challenge, I became a Clerical Officer in the Civil Service; this gave me a thorough grounding in administrative skills. Five years later I returned to work as a dental nurse in the Community Dental Service, eventually moving back into general dental practice.

It was in 1992 that I decided to return to education and study psychology and business management. At this time I also worked part-time as project coordinator for a counselling service for young people and their families. When I had completed my studies, I was asked by Stuart Hawkins, Dental Advisor to Birmingham FHSA, to write a training programme to introduce management skills to senior dental receptionists. This programme was well received and in 1996 was accredited as the BTEC Professional Diploma in Dental Practice Management. In addition to this award I have written BTEC qualifications for dental receptionists: the BTEC Advanced Award in Dental Reception, and, for care coordinators, the BTEC Advanced Award in Dental Patient Education.

Over the past 20 years I have worked closely with many practices, helping them to realise the potential of their teams and compete in the increasingly business-focused world of dentistry. My work has included writing monthly articles for dental journals, making presentations to dental associations, independent dentists and deanery groups, and delivering workshop, in-house and home-learning versions of my BTEC qualifications.

During 2001, in response to requests from student receptionists studying for the BTEC Advanced Award in Dental Reception, along with four of my fellow tutors working for the Dental Resource Company I became a founder member of the British Dental Receptionists Association, formed to give receptionists a voice in the dental community.

If you would like to contact me directly or learn more about what I do, e-mail me at glenys@dental-resource.com or visit the DRC website at www.dental-resource.com.

Special Acknowledgements

Writing this book for dental administrators was an enormous undertaking, which made huge demands upon my time, skills and dedication and those of my family, friends and colleagues whose help and support have been vast and generously given.

Many thanks are due to Caroline Holland who proofread drafts of the text and who, in her thoughts and feedback on the content, gave me the benefit of her extensive knowledge of the world of dentistry. I thank my daughter Gemma, who is my co-director in the Dental Resource Company and has kept the business running whilst I have been otherwise engaged; she has also taken many of the photographs included in the book. Thanks also go to Anita Maniak and Sue Surbey, successive Chairmen of the British Dental Receptionists Association, for their support and input, and to Heidi Cresswell, one of the DRC course tutors who has always been ready to help. Thanks also go to all those dental professionals who have shared their stories with me.

Introduction

Over the past 10 years, governmental measures to modernise health services have recognised a need for more clinicians. In the absence of sufficient numbers of qualified dentists, measures have been developed to train and register the vastly under-used dental care professionals so that they may play a more active role in patient care. Dental nurse radiography and sedation qualifications are just two examples of how dental nurses with adequate training and supervision are already contributing to patient care.

Expanded qualifications and duties for dental nurses will lift their status. However, since there are only so many working hours in the day, when new clinical duties are included other non-clinical duties will have to be taken away. So the expanded role of dental nurses is likely to see the end of the nurse-receptionist role. Many dental employers have recognised that the skills and aptitude required to be a good clinical dental nurse are not necessarily the same skills required to be a good administrator. It therefore becomes possible to develop receptionists with the focus on marketing and customer care skills rather than on clinical skills. In this way practices build up teams made up of individuals each of whom brings complementary skills.

This book has been written with the aim of going some way towards providing background information for those new to dentistry. At the same time it provides additional information on and insight into dental administration and management skills for qualified dental care professionals and dentists.

Section 1
Overview of Dental
Care Administration

Chapter 1
Understanding the Culture
of Dental Care

History of the non-clinical dental team

Teamwork is an essential part of modern dentistry and critical to the provision of high quality dental care. Over recent years, the team roles of dental care professionals (DCPs) have been redefined, with registrable qualifications introduced to ensure whole team professionalism and dental treatments and services focused upon the patient's best interests. More recently the profession has consulted members of the representative groups for DCPs when groundbreaking decisions are to be made.

Before gaining recognition as a profession in its own right, dentistry was considered as a branch of the medical profession. Under the terms of the Medical Act of 1858 Queen Victoria granted a charter to the Royal College of Surgeons to award licences in dentistry. Two years later, 43 candidates passed the first examination to receive the Licentiate of Dental Surgery.

In 1878 the first Dentists Act provided for a register to be kept by the General Medical Council. Until this point there had been no requirement for those carrying out acts of dentistry to hold recognised qualifications. Barber surgeons and blacksmiths frequently extracted teeth in public places with little regard for hygiene or patient care. This changed in 1921 when, to protect the public, a new Dentists Act was introduced under which all 'acts of dentistry' were limited to dentists qualified and registered with the professional lead body.

The next significant milestone for the dental profession was the introduction of the National Health Service in 1948. At this time the majority of dentists worked alone, often from part of their own home converted into a dental surgery. In 1948 the range of treatments delivered by general dental practitioners (GDPs) was limited, with complex procedures being referred to a dental hospital.

At this time, most dentists preferred to mix their own materials. Since air turbines were yet to be invented, a simple saliva ejector was sufficient to keep the treatment area dry. The only assistance dentists required was in the form of someone to answer the doorbell, book appointments as patients left (very few people had a telephone so the phone was not a consideration) and complete the NHS paperwork. In many cases the dentist's wife, or the daughter of a well-off family (who were hoping that their daughter would find a professional husband through her work), fulfilled these duties. In this way, the earliest receptionist role was created.

In the 1950s new generations of dental equipment were developed, in particular the high-speed drills that became standard equipment by the 1960s. Belt-driven drills were replaced by air-driven, water-cooled, high-speed drills. As a result of the water coolants that accompanied this equipment it was necessary for someone to work alongside the dentist to remove excess water for the patient's comfort and to keep the operating area dry. By the late 1950s in some avant-garde, high-tech practices, the four-handed style of dentistry was growing in popularity.

By the late 1960s dentistry was experiencing a period of rapid change. As a result, the role of support staff began to change. A new trend emerged for dentists to work in multi-practitioner practices. At the same time more and more patients were contacting dental practices by telephone. This meant that one-person assisting was no longer adequate. There was a need for someone to work chairside while someone else answered the telephone, managed the appointment book and collected patients' payments. Under these conditions the multi-skilled nurse-receptionist role came into its own in the delivery of patient care.

Another wave of change began in the early 1990s, leading to the development of non-clinical skills. This was driven primarily by two factors: computerisation and patient demands. Computer skills were needed to enable dental businesses to achieve best value from their considerable investment in equipment, and meanwhile non-clinical client care skills were essential as the service aspect of the National Health Service came to the fore. The surgery role also became more involved, with an increased range of skills, knowledge and qualifications being required in order to provide higher quality dental care.

A further impact of the changes of the 1990s was the development of another team role: the practice manager. The number of practice managers in post has grown rapidly since 1992 and continues to grow. The impetus for this is the massive and far-reaching changes in the delivery of primary dental care services, including initiatives such as Clinical Governance and continuous changes in general and employment law. Today, management decisions previously taken by governing authorities on matters such as fee scales and the availability of services are being managed in house, sometimes with little or no guidance. This creates a substantial amount of extra work. Clinically trained practitioners find that running a small business places enormous demands upon their time and resources. As management tasks are not revenue generating, it represents a drain on practice resources. A practice manager is essential to oversee the tactical management of the practice. To fulfil this role, practice managers need a good knowledge of how the practice works and of the needs of both the team and patients.

The practice manager role is still developing, as is the structure of the dental profession. With substantial changes in business aspects of dentistry, the role of practice manager will continue to develop. A whole range of opportunities for the development of the practice manager role are available as a result of corporate dentistry, government policy on Clinical Governance and the increased professional status for DCP groups.

Today's DCPs are highly skilled and, increasingly, highly qualified dental professionals. However, the skills and aptitude required to be a good nurse are not wholly the same as those needed to be an equally good receptionist. The nurse-receptionist role is evolving into two different and highly skilled DCP roles. With the introduction of mandatory dental nurse qualifications, practices may question the deployment of qualified nurses on the reception desk, carrying out work for which qualifications are optional.

Patients are becoming increasingly vocal about their care and treatment. Recent cases brought before the General Dental Council have highlighted issues such as informed consent. Patients are asking questions more often and should be provided with accurate and appropriate responses. The practice manager can ensure that responses are initiated by clinicians and standardised amongst the team.

Options for Change, a government initiative for the 21st century, has completely rewritten the way in which NHS dentistry is to be provided in this country. The financial structure of dentists' payments and patient charges has also been completely redefined.

Likewise, we can expect that the practice manager's role will change as developments occur within the profession, in tandem with changing legislation and increasing patient awareness and expectations. It is an evolving role and will be shaped by all manner of demands as determined by the changing face of dentistry.

On reflection we can see that dental health care has changed dramatically over the last century and is continuing to evolve. As a result, yet another role is emerging, that of the care coordinator. This role will enable dentists to offer a full range of patient education services, with the knowledge that their patients can make informed choices of the treatment options available to them. The care coordinator role will be an important step in the continuing development of dental care.

The ethos and ethics of dental care

Ethos

In the earliest recorded accounts, dentistry is described as a healing art. Advances throughout the 20th century changed the profession dramatically and created today's culture of dental care, and today modern dentistry is an exact, high-tech science. Before becoming a self-regulated profession dentistry had its share of amusing folk remedies, colourful quacks and cults. Now dentists must observe the highest ethical standards by placing patients' interests first and acting to protect them.

Historically, most health-care professions have focused on curative care. Dentistry was one of the first health-care professions to focus on prevention and patient education, aiming to create awareness of the causes of dental problems and to enable patients to make lifestyle changes to prevent dental disease. Today, most general medical practitioners now offer their patients regular health assessments and lifestyle checks, taking an approach tried and tested within the dental profession for decades.

The ethos of modern dentistry developed throughout the last century, guided by successive versions of the Dentists Act. The Dentists Act of 1921 was a milestone in the profession's development. This Act ended an apprenticeship system where both qualified and unqualified dentists and medical practitioners shared the practice of dentistry. William Guy, who introduced this Act, led the drive to stop dental care being delivered by unqualified dentists. He was conscious of the need to protect the public from the dangers of dental treatments performed by unqualified practitioners and devoted his energies to arousing his colleagues from their lethargy and persuading them that legislation prohibiting unqualified practice was absolutely essential for the protection of the public.

The 1921 Act made sure that only registered and qualified dentists were permitted to practise. Since then, a whole range of laws, standards and regulations have been introduced to shape the profession. Other milestones in the development of the dental profession were the introduction of the National Health Service in 1948, and the establishment of the General Dental Council (GDC) in 1956.

Ethics

The GDC's role is to protect patients and regulate the dental team. They protect patients by promoting confidence in dental professionals through the enforcement of ethical standards of practice and conduct. Adherence to a formally agreed set of values is a fundamental aspect of professionalism. The concept of ethical codes specifying standards of behaviour can be tracked back as far as Moses and the Ten Commandments.

Early Grecian civilization is recognised as the birthplace of western ethics. In particular, the teaching of Socrates challenged the right of the strong to oppress the weak, and taught that the strong should uphold the rights of the weak. This was not readily accepted in early Greek society, and in around 400BC Socrates was put to death for 'corrupting the youth of Athens'. Socrates angered the authorities of the day by urging individuals to make reasoned distinctions between what is morally right and what is in their own best interests.

The French philosopher Descartes is considered to be the father of modern western ethics. In his book *Le Monde*, published in 1633, he aimed to 'encourage all who had good sense to think for themselves' and he offered guiding principles and a moral code on which to base thinking, as follows.

Guiding principles

(1) Accept nothing as true that is not self-evident.
(2) Divide problems into their simplest parts.
(3) Solve problems by proceeding from the simple to the complex.
(4) Check and re-check the reasoning.

Moral code

(1) Obey local customs and laws.
(2) Make decisions based on the best evidence.
(3) Change desires, rather than trying to change the world.
(4) Always seek the truth.

Although lifestyles and moral standards have changed considerably since 1633, these guiding principles still provide a basis for building trust and respect.

The GDC publishes ethical guidance for the dental profession and sets guiding principles in the following six key principles of ethical practice.

(1) Put patients' interests first and act to protect them. This principle sets out the responsibility of GDC registrants to work within the scope of their knowledge and keep accurate patient records.
(2) Respect patients' dignity and choices. Here the requirement to treat patients with equality and dignity and give them all the information required to make decisions is outlined.
(3) Protect patients' confidential information. This sets the standard for the use and disclosure of information held about patients and outlines the circumstances under which such information can be disclosed.
(4) Co-operate with other members of the dental team and other health-care colleagues in the interests of patients. Protocols for communications between health-care professionals for the best interests of patients are defined.
(5) Maintain professional knowledge and competence. Dental professionals should keep their knowledge, skills and professional performance under continuous review and identify their limitations as well as their strengths.
(6) Be trustworthy. Dental professionals should act fairly and honestly in all their professional and personal dealings.

Maintaining acceptable standards of behaviour for each of these 'principles' requires every member of the dental team to be fully aware of their role and responsibilities. Guidance is in place to provide clear and detailed definitions and guidance on dental team working.

You can find the most up-to-date information and advice for dental professionals on the GDC website, www.gdc-uk.org.

Dental reception skills

The role of the dental receptionist has changed considerably over recent years. Numerous influences have shaped the role of receptionist as it is today, including public expectations and developments within the dental profession. Today's receptionist needs to be able to draw upon a wide range of skills, some originating from the service sector and others from the health-care sector. In most cases receptionists develop their skills basis from a mixture of formal qualifications and hands-on experience.

The reception is usually the first point of contact patients have with the practice and is the 'shop window' of the practice. Careful consideration should be given to the appearance of the reception area and the reception staff, who should be smartly presented in office wear rather than nurses' uniforms which can be misleading unless reception staff are doubly qualified as nurses.

The role of receptionist goes beyond the immediately obvious. The receptionist is the crucial link between the public and the practice team. Patients' comfort and well-being should be of prime concern to the receptionist. Patients report that waiting for and uncertainty about treatments increase their anxiety. The receptionist should be aware of how patients are feeling and behaving, and should always appear calm and confident. Patients will often reflect the attitude of the receptionist, so reception staff should take the lead when interacting with patients.

It is not only patients who become stressed in the practice: colleagues too can feel under pressure and so taking time to consider how other people are feeling can go a long way to reducing workplace stress. When the appointment book runs late, stress comes to the forefront. Here the receptionist should be aware of the need to liaise effectively between the surgery and the patient, keeping everyone informed and maintaining good will. A good receptionist learns to judge the mood of patients, dentists and work colleagues.

When speaking to patients over the telephone, the receptionist should sound friendly and efficient. It is important to maintain a positive tone. Your practice should set telephone protocols to reflect the ideals of the practice, which are observed by all members of the team when answering the telephone.

An important aspect of the practice is the atmosphere surrounding the reception area. Reception working areas should be kept uncluttered and tidy at all times, as this shows competence and control of your work environment. This calls for methodical working systems, which are vital to add professionalism to administrative services. Learning to work under pressure comes with experience.

The role of the receptionist will vary from practice to practice. The team role of the receptionist is outlined by the British Dental Receptionists Association in broad terms as follows:

'As part of the practice team, to assist in the provision of dental care services . . . . To embrace the organisation, implementation and delivery of dental services by developing patient care procedures to ensure maximum contribution to the practice's profitability, in line with GDC guidelines and practice policies.'

This is carried out through the following tasks:

- Open and close the practice each working day.
- Welcome patients and visitors and direct them to appropriate waiting areas.
- Notify providers (dentist or hygienist) of each patient's arrival.
- Review adherence to schedule and remind the provider, and inform patients of excessive delays.
- Anticipate patients' anxieties.
- Answer patients' questions.
- Arrange appointments in person or by telephone.
- Enter and retrieve patient records.
- Send out recalls.
- Receive and redirect all incoming telephone calls as appropriate.
- Operate the central paging and music system.
- Operate the computer system in accordance with legal and ethical guidelines.
- Monitor the hazard warning systems and notify the appropriate person of occurrences.
- Sell sundry products at patients' requests.
- Calculate and collect patient charges.
- Note feedback from patients.
- Complete NHS claims.
- Respond to emergencies in line with practice policy.
- Participate in professional development activities.
- Attend regular staff meetings.

Perform these and other related duties necessary to maintain a high standard of patient care with due regard for patient confidentiality.

The person specification

The receptionist's job description should be agreed and written down and should be reviewed as part of the appraisal process. Any areas in which improvements are required can be addressed and an action plan agreed to strengthen areas of underperformance. The receptionist plays an extremely important role in ensuring the smooth running of the practice. Because it is vital that work is carried out to the highest possible standard, employers are advised to look for the following skills when recruiting reception staff.

To begin with the receptionist must be organised and efficient. This will result in work being carried out in an effective and efficient manner. Employers know the effects of a badly run reception; it will have repercussions throughout the practice. An organised reception also looks more professional to patients, and may make nervous patients feel at ease whereas a chaotic workplace appears unprofessional and may increase their anxiety.

Good timekeeping is also essential. The receptionist needs to be on the premises in good time to greet the first patients of the session.

Receptionists should be observant. It is important to monitor the comings and goings of patients and to keep an eye on the waiting room. If a patient has been waiting for a long time, an apology must be made and the situation should be brought to the attention of the dentist.

Good communication skills are an essential attribute. If communication is lacking between team members, it often means things get forgotten, missed or not done properly. It is equally important for the dental receptionist to be able to communicate with the patients. At times this will involve using a sympathetic caring manner, whereas at other times assertiveness will be required. Nervous patients need a reassuring tone of voice to help calm their nerves, but difficult issues or complaints may need to be dealt with using a more assertive approach. Speaking in a clear voice is very important so that people can fully understand what you are saying. Listening can be just as important as speaking, and if a message needs passing on it needs to retain its meaning enough to make sense to the person for whom it is intended.

Good administrative skills are needed in order to ensure that all reception duties are prioritised and completed with competence. At times the receptionist will be required to make decisions within the framework of the practice rules, and should be confident enough to do so.

Being computer literate is also an advantage as most dental practices now rely on computer systems for booking appointments and typing referral letters.

Customer care skills are vital, especially a friendly disposition which must be retained even at the busiest of times and when working under pressure.

To ensure patients' dental experiences are positive, receptionists must have the following skills and abilities:

Communication	Being comfortable communicating with all types of people.
Empathy	Being able to see matters from the patient's point of view.
Organisation	Ability to deliver streamlined and friendly services.
Language	Ability to speak clearly using appropriate language.

With these skills and abilities in place, receptionists project the image of being confident and competent dental professionals who take pride in their work.

Practice management skills

In today's dental practices, everyone needs to be committed to the concept of 'whole team professionalism'. This means each member of the dental team needs to have a working knowledge of the principles of professionalism, leading to adherence to a set of values comprising both a formally agreed-upon code of conduct and the informal expectations of colleagues and society. The key values are to act in patients' best interests, with obligations for the health needs of society. When each person in the team is fully committed to these standards, the role of practice manager is straightforward.

In many cases, managers are finding workers increasingly difficult to manage, especially those who do not respect rank or rules and are more concerned about themselves, their families and the deals they can make for their own benefit than with loyalty or commitment to standards of professionalism. At times managers feel they are in a stressful tug-of-war. On one side are the demands of professionalism, and on the other side the demands of employees, added to which they are continuously trying to define their level of authority. The title of practice manager does not guarantee respect just as drawing up a policy does not ensure implementation, and delegation of work does not ensure the desired results.

Never before have the skills of management been so frequently studied and defined as over recent years, resulting in strongly contested debate over the merits of the hands-on versus hands-off management approaches. Managers should be alert to the fact that, where the hands-off approach is used, the result may be a severe case of undermanagement with resulting deterioration in worker–employer relationships and a lowering of work standards. When asked, managers who preferred this approach claim they are 'empowering' their people by remaining hands off. Although nobody wants to be micro-managed, the feeling that the boss is breathing down your neck is claustrophobic. It is just as hazardous as the hands-off approach when it is used as a cloaking device for the manager's shortfalls in the basic skills required to focus and motivate the team.

Undermanagement results when managers fail to keep informed about the details of their team members' tasks and responsibilities, and they neglect to provide clear direction and support or to hold individuals accountable for their performance. Failure to provide these management basics leads to a downward spiral which is devastating to both the credibility of managers and the motivation of employees.

HOT management

The opposite approach to hands-off management is hands-on management. The term 'HOT management' is used to describe a hands-on transactional management style, which requires managers to be:

Informed: Fully aware of both the legal and ethical obligations placed upon dental professionals, and understanding their teams' challenges and triumphs.

Comfortable: With their role and justly confident in their management competence, and with adequate support mechanisms for managers and the teams they manage.

Understanding: Having empathy for the needs of both patients and employees, leading to recognition of people's problems and achievements.

Relaxed: In their approach to personnel management, using a calm 'can-do' approach supported by policies and protocols to provide an equitable working environment.

Confident: When dealing with difficult people and circumstances.

Leaders: Effective leaders give clear direction, and set standards by example whilst supporting all the team to meet those standards.

In touch: With team members and aware of each person's value to the team.

Sociable: Networking with colleagues in the dental community, sharing ideas and experiences, and considering them as allies, not competitors.

Innovative: Not stuck in a rut; prepared to make carefully thought-out changes.

Successful: Business success brings rewards on all levels; 'work smarter', making best use of the team's skills and enjoying the rewards.

The nature of management lies between a science and an art. This requires managers to have good aptitude for the objective scientific skills such as managing income and expenditure, organising practicalities and setting the policies, procedures and protocols to create equitable, consistent and robust workplace environments. In addition they need a range of soft management skills such as providing pastoral care to build loyalty, motivation and a sense of belonging into the team. On their own, excellence in only one of these types of skills leads to poor team performance: good management is a balance of both aptitudes.

Specific duties

The specific duties of practice managers will vary from practice to practice. In its broadest sense the team role of practice manager can be described as follows:

The practice manager will be responsible for the running, design and implementation of agreed administrative, financial, marketing and personnel management systems on a continually developing basis, working as part of the practice team to assist in the provision of high-quality dental care services to our patients. The practice manager must further the practice's objectives for the provision of quality dental services in line with the practice's ethos and with GDC guidelines.

Financial management
- Check invoices and pay minor creditors in line with company guidance.
- Liaise with the employer on salary enquiries.
- Supervise all practice banking procedures.
- Clarify terms of business to clients and thus reduce incidents of bad debt and failed appointments.
- Ensure that relevant payment claims are made and reconciled.
- Streamline processes and reduce the amount of clinical surgery time used for non-clinical tasks.

Personnel management
- Assist with recruitment, training and Induction procedures.
- Encourage, motivate and mentor staff in line with practice policy.
- Deploying of staff, maintaining appropriate staffing levels at all times in line with practice policy.
- Maintain records and report to the employer on staff sickness and holidays.
- Operate the staff discipline and grievance system.
- Maintain a team culture of respect and equitability.
- Organise and record staff training.
- Coordinate arrangements for staff appraisals.
- Organise and participate in staff meetings.

Practice development
- Monitor the appointment books.
- Promote the image of the practice in ways consistent with practice policy.
- Monitor client feedback.
- Design administrative systems within the remit of your position.
- Maintain NHS and Independent/Dental Complaints Service (DCS) complaints procedures.
- Maintain referrals system.
- Perform other related duties to maintain a high standard of patient care.
- Work with the lead dentists to monitor compliance with Clinical Governance consistent with practice guidelines.
- Oversee the implementation of the practice business and marketing plan.

General
- Arrange promotional events to raise the profile of the practice within the local community.
- Review and streamline procedures.
- Liaise with suppliers and representatives on behalf of the practice.
- Ensure compliance with health and safety legislation, the Disability Discrimination Act, and fire safety law.
- Oversee maintenance of all practice equipment.
- Inspect all parts of the practice weekly; record and report deficiencies or malfunctions in line with practice policy.
- Supervise security of the building and alarm system, and maintain a list of key holders.
- Maintain the first aid box, accident book and other such compliance measures.

Patient services
- Ensure the efficient operation of the patient recall system.
- Ensure the effective operation of patient complaints procedures.
- Respond to patient queries in a polite and professional manner.
- Ensure sufficient high quality information is available for patients at all times.

Practice manager person specification

Essential attributes
- Must hold appropriate qualifications, fitness to practice certification, Criminal Records Bureau clearance.
- Computer literacy.
- Excellent communication skills.
- Customer interface experience.
- Proactive approach.
- Previous experience of working in a supervisory role within the health-care sector.
- 'Can do' attitude.

Desirable attributes
- Recent experience of working within a team in a general dental practice.
- Experience of communicating non-clinical terms of dental care to colleagues and patients.
- Team player with strong relationship-building skills with colleagues and patients.
- Marketing or sales experience.
- Diligence.
- Motivation and keenness to further their professional development.

Salary
To British Dental Practice Managers Association pay scale.

The practice manager role is still developing, as also is the structure of the dental profession. With substantial changes in the business aspects of dentistry, the role of practice manager will continue to develop, offering managers a wide range of opportunities for personal and professional growth.

Chapter 2
Who's Who in the Dental Team

The team

Over recent years the roles and qualifications for dental professionals have undergone massive changes. As a result careers for dental care professionals (DCPs) are more structured, with the General Dental Council specifying the curriculum for registrable qualifications for all of the dental team rather than solely for dentists. The curricular framework in which the knowledge, skills and aptitudes required for whole team professionalism are defined ensures DCPs are equipped to play expanded roles in the provision of high-quality dental services.

Teamwork is the essence of modern dentistry. Dental teams are made up of groups of dental professionals, each contributing their specific skills and expertise. For teams to work well, each person must have a clear understanding of where they fit into their team. When practices produce a company structure diagram as shown in Figure 2.1, the hierarchy is clarified and each person can focus on fulfilling their team roles as follows.

Dentists

There are around 27 000 dentists working in general practice in the UK. Between 1948, when the National Health Service was established, and the early 1990s, most dentists worked as independent contractors for the Department of Health, providing National Health Service (NHS) treatment. Recently, many dentists resigned either wholly or in part from the NHS because of their dissatisfaction with the terms of service and remuneration.

Many dental practices are small, owner-run businesses, requiring dentists to develop a range of business management skills to ensure the viability of their practices. Some dentists choose not to take on this additional role and opt to work for corporates; these are dental companies registered with the General Dental Council to provide dental care to the public. Dentists working for dental corporates provide dental care, and the corporate employs managers to manage the business.

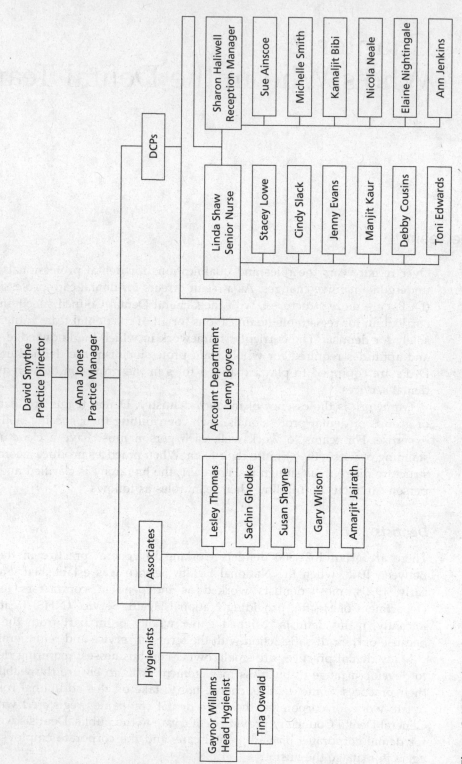

Figure 2.1 Our dental care team.

There is a shortage of dentists in the UK. In some areas the shortage of dental care provision is critical and health authorities have opened Dental Access Centres employing salaried dentists to provide emergency care.

To provide patients with the highest quality of care, dentists work alongside dental nurses, hygienists, therapists, technicians, practice managers and receptionists.

Qualifications

Fourteen dental schools in the UK offer the five-year courses leading to either BDS or BChD qualifications. Once qualified, dentists must register with the General Dental Council, the profession's governing body. After graduating, most dentists choose to work in general dental practice and undertake a vocational training programme during which they work under the supervision of an experienced dentist appointed as their vocational trainer and mentor.

Once qualified, dentists are required to commit to their continued professional development by meeting criteria for lifelong learning set by the GDC. Practitioners must provide evidence of having met these criteria to renew their annual registration, without which they are not permitted to carry out acts of dentistry.

Dental nurses

Dental nurses play an essential role in the smooth running of the treatment room by assisting dentists, therapists and hygienists in the provision of dental treatments. With detailed knowledge of treatment procedures, nurses make materials and instruments readily available to clinicians as required and provide suction to keep the operating area clear and dry for the clinician to work in and for the patient's comfort. Nurses are responsible for ensuring the patient's comfort and safety during their appointment.

Before each appointment, the dental nurse prepares the treatment room. During assessment visits (examinations), the dental nurse records the dentist's findings in the patient's records. When the patient leaves the treatment room, the dental nurse performs stringent cross-infection control measures, decontaminating clinical areas and sterilising all of the instruments. Some dental nurses also work on reception or do a variety of administrative tasks.

Qualifications

In general dental practices, the initial training for new dental nurses is conducted by dentists and senior nurses. To gain qualifications, student nurses must enrol with a training provider who will provide evening classes, day release or home learning tuition towards recognised qualifications.

Before registration of dental nurses, employers decided upon whether or not dental nurses were formally qualified. As a result, although some dental nurses were qualified and enrolled on the Voluntary Register of Dental Nurses, those who were trained only by their employers do not hold a formal qualification. Only nurses holding an approved qualification can be registered. However, there will be a two-year window in which dental nurses not holding a recognised qualification can apply to the GDC, who will assess whether or not their training and experience equip them for registration. At the end of this two-year 'transitional period', only dental nurses with recognised qualifications can become registered.

The main qualifications for dental nurses are the National Certificate in Dental Nursing or the National Vocational Qualification in Oral Health Care. Dental hospitals also run their own dental nurse training programmes and their own certificates of proficiency in dental nursing.

New career paths are now open to qualified and registered dental nurses. Many dental nurses qualify as dental radiographers, studying for the Certificate in Dental Radiography, a qualification offered jointly by the Dental Nurses Examining Board, the College of Radiography (COR) and the British Society of Dental and Maxillofacial Radiology (BSDMFR). Having completed this course nurses are qualified to take dental x-rays.

Nurses interested in oral health promotion can take a BTEC qualification in oral health education and work as a health educator, concentrating on preventative care and the effects of smoking and alcohol upon oral health. Other career options for qualified dental nurses include training to be an orthodontic nurse, special care nurse, or care coordinator.

Hygienists

There are around 3900 dental hygienists in the UK. Their role is concerned with patient education and promoting oral health as a part of a preventative approach to dental disease. After a dentist has made an assessment of the patient's treatment needs, if necessary a scale and polish appointment is made with the hygienist who provides a thorough cleaning of the teeth and gums and advice on how to carry out effective home care procedures such as regular flossing and careful brushing. Most patients benefit from a six-monthly visit to the hygienist to maintain good gum health. When patients show early signs of gum conditions such as gingivitis, the dentist will refer them to a hygienist for a course of treatment. Hygienists are also able to apply fluoride treatments and fissure sealants, which protect children's teeth from decay.

Because of the low numbers of hygienists in the UK, some practices who would ideally like to employ one are not able to do so and therefore dentists carry out routine cleaning and provide oral hygiene advice themselves. Others employ an oral health educator or care coordinator to provide patients with the necessary skills to maintain their oral health.

Qualifications

Many dental hygienists first qualify as dental nurses and then apply to a school of dental hygiene to further their careers. There are two recognised qualifications for hygienists. These are the Diploma in Dental Hygiene and the combined Diploma in Dental Therapy. With the expansion of DCP roles in general dental practices, the hygienist role and qualification continue to develop.

Hygienists must be qualified and registered with the GDC to practise in the UK. The full-time training courses for dental hygienists run for two years. Schools of dental hygiene are attached to dental teaching hospitals. Competition for the few places available each year is very fierce.

Dental therapists

There are currently about 370 dental therapists working in the UK. This number is expected to grow following a change in the law, which allows them to work in general dental practice. Therapists carry out certain clinical procedures such as simple fillings, extractions and fitting crowns. They can also take impressions (moulds) and dental x-rays, treat patients under sedation and provide injections.

When the dental therapist role was first introduced in the UK, they worked solely in the community dental service (school clinics). A dentist would carry out an initial examination and then certain treatments were referred to a therapist, working under the supervision of a dentist.

Over recent years the role of the therapist has been expanded and dentists in general dental practice are allowed to employ therapists to deliver specified treatments. Additional dental therapy training schools are being opened to train more therapists to work in the UK. Dental hygienists are able to top up their qualifications; by taking extra training they can qualify as dental therapists.

Qualifications

Dental therapists must be qualified and enrolled with the GDC in order to practise in the UK. Qualifications approved for enrolment include the Diploma in Dental Therapy or Combined Diploma in Hygiene and Dental Therapy (awarded by schools of dental hygiene and therapy) and a BSc (Hons) in dental hygiene and dental therapy.

Practice managers

The role of the practice manager is relatively new to dental practice and developed during the 1990s as dental practices became more business focused. Responsible for the day-to-day smooth running of the practice, practice managers oversee relevant legal, personnel and business issues, thus enabling dentists to concentrate on clinical matters.

Many practice managers began their careers in dentistry as dental nurses, receptionists or hygienists, although in some cases dentists employ practice managers from a non-dental, management background to expand the range of skills within the team.

The practice manager role varies from practice to practice, often including financial management tasks such as book-keeping, payroll, budgeting, predicting and managing cash flow and preparing financial reports. Personnel management duties include recruiting, training and managing staff, and administrative duties include the design and implementation of procedures such as referral systems and NHS claims. Increasingly today's practice managers are responsible for the maintenance and development of the practice's IT systems as well as for handling practice promotion and patient feedback schemes.

Qualifications

Although many in the profession categorise practice managers with DCPs, because their role is non-clinical they are not required to hold a recognised qualification or to register with the GDC. The skills and knowledge required to effectively manage a dental practice are such that the qualifications available in dental practice management are at NVQ level 4 or above. The most established qualification is the BTEC Professional Diploma in Dental Practice Management, holders of which are entitled to use the letters Cert DPM after their name.

Receptionists

The role of dental receptionist has changed considerably over recent years. Receptionists need to be expert in a range of skills drawn from the service and health-care sectors, requiring a mixture of formal and hands-on training and experience to meet the needs of patients and their colleagues in the dental team. As much of the receptionist's work is performed in the view of patients, methodical working systems are important and add to the practice's image of professionalism.

The role of receptionists goes beyond the immediately obvious. Receptionists are the vital link between the public and the practice team. As such they play a key role in marketing the practice, so consideration should be given to their appearance and approach to patients and colleagues.

The comfort and well-being of patients are of prime concern to the receptionist. Many patients are anxious when visiting the dentist and their anxiety is increased by unexpectedly long waiting times and by uncertainty about what will happen in the treatment room. Receptionists should be alert to how patients are feeling and behaving and always remain calm and confident. It is not only patients who can become stressed; as everyday workplace stresses come to the fore, receptionists should be aware that their role requires them to liaise between the team and the patient, keeping everyone informed and maintaining goodwill.

When speaking to patients over the telephone, the receptionist should be friendly and efficient. It is important to handle patients in a positive way. There should be telephone protocols in place for the practice, to be followed by any team member when speaking to patients on the phone. Learning to work under pressure comes with experience. A good receptionist learns to judge the mood of patients, dentists and team work colleagues.

Qualifications

Like the practice manager the receptionist has a non-clinical role and is not required to hold recognised qualifications or to register with the GDC. Training and qualifications are at the employer's discretion. In many cases training is delivered in house. The British Dental Receptionists Association recommends that, following six months' hands-on experience in practice, members take the BTEC Advanced Award in Dental Reception to gain a good grounding in the appropriate knowledge and skills for receptionists. The qualification acknowledges students' existing knowledge and skills, and facilitates the development and application of formal administration and reception skills. The course has been developed to meet the needs of both new and experienced receptionists, irrespective of whether their previous experience is in dentistry or any other area of health care.

Care coordinators

The role of care coordinator is the most recent addition to the dental team. This role was developed to reinforce the work of the clinician. After the patient has been seen and diagnosed by a dentist, the care coordinator can spend time discussing treatment options to help patients make informed choices about treatment options and their costs. In busy dental practices patients often feel they cannot ask all of the questions they would ideally like to. Care coordinators are communicators who spend time establishing patients' perceived dental needs and showing them how they can be met with the range of care options now available to patients, empowering patients to make genuinely informed choices. The introduction of the care coordinator role into dental practices offers a highly effective win–win approach to patient care.

The skills required to work effectively as care coordinator combine a knowledge of sociology, psychology, communication and ethical selling. Most care coordinators are experienced members of dental teams, either nurses or receptionists, who participate in further studies over six months to develop their insight into patient perspectives in order to provide themselves with all the information they need.

Qualifications

In June 2001 the Dental Resource Company developed a qualification for dental care coordinators, the BTEC Advanced Award in Dental Care Education, to enable practices to reap the benefits of a whole new approach to non-clinical client care. The role of care coordinator is becoming increasingly common in dental teams across the UK, where there is a real desire to empower patients to make informed decisions about their oral health. This is achieved by actively assisting patients to understand their prescribed treatment choices in terms of the value rather than simply the cost of each option. Training can be delivered in house, or through home learning or workshops. See www.dental-resource.com.

The dental trade

The dental trade consists of the companies providing goods and services to the dental profession including manufacturers, wholesalers, distributors and service providers. Some dental supply houses send their representatives out to practices to collect orders, whereas others prefer to trade online or through call centres. Manufacturers employ reps to introduce new products to dentists by taking samples and showing dentists the results of scientific trials carried out on new materials.

Competition within the distribution sector of the dental trade is fierce and it is possible for practices to negotiate some very favourable discounts by putting all of their purchases through the same distributor.

The dental trade supports dental teams in numerous ways. These include providing generous sponsorship for dental conferences, funding professional awards, such as the Probe Awards, and providing grants and bursaries for individuals to study for additional qualifications. From their point of view such initiatives provide them with good publicity and build enduring relationships with current and future customers.

The British Dental Trade Association (BDTA) holds a trade exhibition called Dental Showcase every 18 months. This major event in the dental calendar draws exhibitors from every aspect of the dental trade. It runs from Thursday to Saturday and attracts many thousands of visitors from every part of the profession. In many practices the whole team attends for team building and professional development.

Qualifications

The Dental Industry Training Institute (DITI) is the training arm of the BDTA. Under the Association's Code of Practice, members are responsible for ensuring that their staff has the ongoing experience, product knowledge and ability necessary to perform their duties properly and effectively. This includes effective and timely responses to customers' queries.

As a minimum, all relevant staff should have attained the BDTA Introduction to Dentistry Certificate within two years of commencement of employment with a member. BDTA training courses are available to assist in this process and provide benchmark training standards within the dental industry. The BDTA is also a source of information and advice on training, educational and career issues within the dental industry.

Dental technicians

There are approximately 8000 dental technicians in the UK. Dental technicians are important members of the dental team. They make a wide range of dental prosthetics including crowns, bridges, orthodontic appliances and dentures. Although in most cases technicians work in privately owned commercial laboratories, providing services to practices, dental technicians are an integral part of the dental team working to the written instructions of dentists.

At present some technicians, known as denturists, work outside the law set out in the Dentists Act 1984. They make dentures for members of the public without a clinical assessment by a dentist. The change in legislation aims to protect the public, by ensuring that patients without any natural teeth still have periodical soft tissue examinations carried out by a dentist. Such examinations could potentially identify conditions of the oral tissues that could be successfully treated if identified at an early stage.

Qualifications

Formal qualifications and registration for dental technicians will be introduced through the same legislation that will bring about dental nurse registration. This will enable patients who have been clinically assessed by a dentist to have certain dentures made by a registered clinical dental technician, working from a registered dental laboratory not necessarily sited within a dental practice. This will follow the model established for optical services, where patients are free to choose where they go to purchase spectacles after an eye examination and being given a prescription for lenses.

Historically the main qualification for dental technicians has been a BTEC National in Dental Technology. However, in September 2004, the first foundation degree (fd) for dental technicians was approved and introduced into colleges up and down the country. Development of the foundation degree was undertaken by a consortium from the colleges via a 'hub' at the People's College, Nottingham, in conjunction with De Montfort University, Leicester.

Using college-based learning and effective evidence of structured vocational training provided in the real workplace, the fd provides dental technology education and training. Colleges offer this fd at their own centres, linked to the local employer dental laboratories' work-based training. The fd was developed to match the registrable requirements set by the General Dental Council.

Today more than ever it is vital that everyone in the dental team is highly skilled and qualified to play their role in patient care. Long gone are the days when DCPs simply had a job at the dentists. Today, as dental professionals in their own right, DCPs have careers in dentistry and demonstrate this by maintaining the highest standards of excellence in their work.

Official bodies within dentistry

National Health Service (NHS)

Europe's biggest employer, the National Health Service (NHS), was established with the National Health Service Act in 1946. The NHS provides three tiers of care, primary, secondary and tertiary. Patients can access primary care services on a self-referred basis, by visiting their dentist, GP, pharmacist or optician. Secondary care includes general medical and dental services in hospitals and other locations; these services are provided to patients referred by primary care practitioners. Tertiary care services are highly specialised, such as those delivered in intensive care units or neuro- and thoracic surgery, requiring highly sophisticated technology and facilities.

The NHS was instigated by Aneurin Bevan to provide health-care services free at the point of delivery to those in need, financed by central government. Following a five-year period of national hardship during the Second World War, the NHS was introduced to improve the health of the nation, based on the belief that, as the nation became healthier, demands placed upon the NHS would decrease. In fact, because the NHS has succeeded in keeping people alive longer and has developed new services, demands on the NHS have exceeded original expectations and continue to grow.

The first ten years of the NHS saw very little capital investment. By 1951, cash shortages required the collection of fees from dental and optical patients for false teeth and spectacles to finance ongoing services. This deviation from the original policy of offering treatment free at the point of delivery caused uproar in Parliament and throughout the country. Restructuring of the NHS has been ongoing since the 1950s; in November 2004 the structure shown in Figure 2.2 was introduced, replacing the structure introduced in 2002. Under this structure the NHS is funded from taxation and patients' fees. The Secretary of State for Health decides how funds are distributed throughout the NHS and is accountable to Parliament for performance. The Department of Health is responsible for running and improving the NHS, and works with the following 'at arm's length government bodies' to develop services:

- the Modernisation Agency;
- Executive Agencies;
- Non-executive Agencies;
- Special Health Authorities.

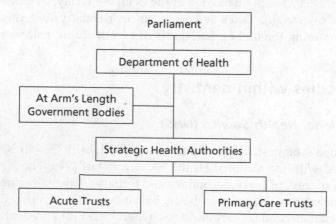

Figure 2.2 Structure of the NHS: England.

Strategic Health Authorities (SHAs)

There are 28 SHAs, which provide links between the Department of Health and the NHS Trusts and Primary Care Trusts (PCTs). Their role is to support and monitor the work of PCTs.

Acute Trusts

These NHS Trusts manage hospitals, making sure that they provide high quality health care and that they spend their money efficiently. They also decide on a strategy for how the hospital will develop so that services improve.

Primary Care Trusts (PCTs)

Primary Care Trusts are the local health organisations responsible for managing local health services. Their role is to ensure that there are enough services for local people. There are 303 PCTs throughout England, each responsible for a specific area. Funding is provided for each PCT from the Department of Health. When you first have a health problem, you turn to a primary care provider such as a dentist, optician or doctor. The PCTs are responsible for all of the providers in their area. Each PCT has three main roles: to improve the health of local people and reduce inequalities in health; to provide effective and responsive local health services; and to commission the best possible services for local people from NHS hospitals. An Executive and a Board make the decisions about how the trust will be run. The Executive is the 'engine room' of the PCT, with responsibility for thinking through how the trust will invest its funds, and sets the policies they will use. The Executive typically consists of up to seven GPs, two nurses, a professional with public health and health promotion experience, and a social services officer. The Board is drawn from the Executive and is typically made up of 11 members consisting of a chairperson, five lay members, a chief executive, a finance director, and three professional members. These professionals tend to be a GP, a nurse and a Clinical Governance director. The Secretary of State appoints the chair and lay members.

General Dental Council (GDC)

General Dental Council

The General Dental Council regulates dental professionals in the UK. Dentists, dental hygienists and dental therapists must hold current registration with the GDC to work within the UK. Dental nurses and dental technicians have been regulated by the GDC since July 2006. All registered dental professionals need to be suitably qualified and to keep up to date through continued professional development (CPD). By law, dentists must do 250 hours of CPD every five years to stay on the GDC's register. In future CPD will be compulsory for all dental professionals on the GDC's registers.

The GDC was established for the protection of the public and fulfils this role by:

- quality-assuring the education and training of dental professionals in the UK;
- maintaining a register of those suitably qualified to perform acts of dentistry;
- re-registering practitioners annually to maintain their eligibility to practise dentistry;
- publishing a register of dental professionals;
- setting standards of dental practice behaviour;
- managing complaints from the public regarding dental professionals' skills, behaviour or health.

The GDC is empowered to act through three statutory committees:

- the Preliminary Proceedings Committee;
- the Professional Conduct Committee;
- the Health Committee.

The GDC's work includes providing information to patients and guidance to the profession to ensure the interests of the public are protected. Members of the public can search the GDC database of registered practitioners by visiting their website, www.gdc-uk.org, as well as being able to make a complaint about a registered dental professional.

Corporate dentistry

The General Dental Council currently has regulatory powers, which extend to the dental bodies corporate. Businesses are required to provide the GDC with annual returns outlining aspects of their businesses. Under the Dentists Act of 1956 the formation of new companies to carry on the business of dentistry was banned, although the 27 already in existence at that time were allowed to remain. Moves have been made to remove this ban, as the GDC does not consider that it plays a role in public protection.

In the mid-1990s interest in existing dental bodies corporate grew considerably. Companies paid six-figure amounts to purchase dental bodies corporate to permit them to go on to purchase practices throughout the UK and form a branded chain of dental care outlets. Corporate chains are managed centrally through a corporate management structure, thus freeing dentists from the burdens of business ownership and of day-to-day practice management.

The professions' initial reaction to the rise of corporates was one of concern. However, with hindsight many would now agree that DBCs have played an important role in the development of dental services over recent years.

Dental Practice Board (DPB)

The Dental Practice Board was set up by the National Health Service Act of 1946 and came into being in 1948, though at that time it was called the Dental Estimates Board. It was created to manage the payment and monitoring of treatment provided under the General Dental Services of the NHS. The Dental Estimates Board was renamed as the Dental Practice Board by the Health and Medicines Act 1988 and continued to be situated at the same Eastbourne site built originally as Temple Grove School but occupied during the war by the National Association of Approved Societies.

The statutory duties of the DPB are:

- considering NHS dental claim forms for prior approval of treatment or for payment;
- preparing monthly payment schedules of fees;
- paying NHS dentists;
- detecting and bringing to the notice of the health bodies (PCTs) any apparent failure by dentists to comply with their terms of service;
- submitting an annual report to the Secretary of State for Health for England and Wales and supplying such statistical or other information relating to the DPB's work as required.

NHS

Business Services Authority

Dental Practice Division

The Dental Practice Board was dissolved on 31 March 2006 when it merged into the NHS Business Services Authority (BSA) as set out in the policy document 'Reconfiguring the Department of Health's Arm's Length Bodies'. As a division of the BSA it will continue to operate payment systems in respect of NHS dentists' contracts and collect data relating to the provisions of NHS dental treatment under the new dental contract introduced on 1 April 2006.

From 1 April 2006 PCTs became responsible for commissioning NHS general dental services and for monitoring the activities of dentists. Practices providing NHS treatment entered into new General Dental Services (nGDS) contracts, with an agreed annual value for the provision of NHS care and an agreed level of activity. The contract value, minus patients' charges, is paid to practices in 12 monthly payments.

Representative bodies

Professional associations have been formed to represent the interests of their members within the dental community. Some groups of dental professionals have the choice of a number of relevant groups and associations. The most prominent representative bodies are as follows.

British Dental Association

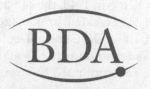

There are a number of professional bodies for dentists. The primary representative body for dentists is the British Dental Association (BDA). The British Dental Association describes itself as the professional association and trade union for dentists in the UK. With over 18 000 qualified members, the majority of the profession have chosen to join. The BDA develops policies to represent dentists working in every sphere, from general practice, through community and hospital settings, to universities and the armed forces.

The BDA aims to get the best for its members, both in terms of practical help through services and products and by ensuring that it is a national player in the development of health-care policy. It provides its members with legal, health and safety, and educational advice as well as influencing government policy in each of the UK's four nations. Their website address is www.bda.org.

British Association of Dental Nurses (BADN)

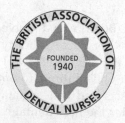

The British Association of Dental Nurses is the UK's only recognised professional association for dental nurses. Membership is open to dental nurses in all areas of dentistry, whether or not they are qualified. The day-to-day administration is carried out at their headquarters in Fleetwood. An elected council of dental nurses runs the BADN, all of whom give their time to further the profession of dental nursing. The BADN represents the interests of dental nurses at all levels of the profession and works with all appropriate organisations – such as the General Dental Council, the National Examining Board for Dental Nurses, and other dental organisations. The BADN organises the Annual BADN Dental Nursing Conference and regular study days, which are open to all members of the dental team.

BADN members enjoy a wide range of membership benefits, ranging from free legal advice to discounts on products and services, insurance and health care, in addition to their quarterly journal *The British Dental Nurses' Journal*. As well as a Regional and Local Group network, BADN has specialist National Groups for dental nurses working in the armed forces, orthodontics, special care, sedation, practice management/reception, and training and assessment. Their website, www.badn.org.uk, has a members-only area with up-to-date information on developments in dental nursing. Members also receive an information CD-rom which can be updated from the members-only area of the website.

British Dental Hygienists' Association

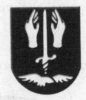

The British Dental Hygienists' Association strives to:

- promote the study of oral health and to provide a consultative body to which reference may be made by public or private bodies for guidance in connection with the dental hygienist profession;
- maintain the honour and interests of the dental hygienist profession;
- represent and safeguard the common interests of members;
- provide opportunities for post-qualification education.

Their website address is www.bhda.org.uk.

British Association of Dental Therapists

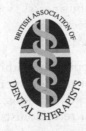

The British Association of Dental Therapists represents dental therapists. Its objectives are:

- to promote the interests and well-being of BADT members;
- to promote co-operation and to provide a channel of communication between the members of the Association;
- to promote the study and advancement of knowledge in the field of work carried out by dental therapists;
- to liaise with other professional bodies;
- to encourage the promotion of oral health in the community.

Their website address is www.badt.org.uk.

British Dental Practice Managers Association

The British Dental Practice Managers Association is the representative body for practice managers. The Association was formed in 1993 by a group of practice managers in Birmingham. The BDPMA has established a national membership and offers support and information for practice managers via a wide range of membership services, a quarterly newsletter, regional meetings and an annual National Conference. Their website address is www.bdpma.org.uk.

British Dental Receptionists' Association

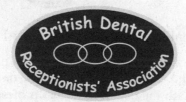

The British Dental Receptionists' Association (BDRA) was formed on 19 January 2002. Previous to this, receptionists were the only group within the dental profession not to have a representative body. The Association was formed to give receptionists a voice within the dental community and to provide guidance to members on pay, conditions and training requirements. The BDRA aims to clarify the developing role of receptionist as the front-of-house representative of dental businesses, with proficiency in the skills of both the health-care and service sectors.

The aims of the BDRA are to:

- define the role of receptionist within the dental team;
- offer opportunities for the development of relevant skills;
- establish benchmark qualifications;
- represent the views of receptionists within the profession;

- provide a channel of communication and interchange of ideas among receptionists;
- provide pay guidelines.

Their website address is www.bdra.org.uk.

British Dental Trade Association

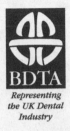

The British Dental Trade Association (BDTA) is a group of manufacturers, wholesalers, distributors and suppliers of products and services to the dental profession who have joined together for their mutual advantage. Members gain access to a range of services designed to benefit them and promote the well-being of the industry as a whole. The BDTA was established in 1923 and today represents the interests of 105 member companies. It is a non-profit making organisation governed by a council of elected representatives, which meets six times a year. The council establishes committees and working groups to carry out marketing, training, editorial and statistical activities. Member companies have opportunities to put forward individuals to participate in the various committees when vacancies arise.

One of the highlights of the dental year is the BDTA Dental Showcase, a trade exhibition drawing dental professionals from throughout the UK.

Their website address is www.bdta.org.uk.

Dental Technicians Association

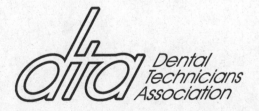

Before 2002 the Dental Technicians' Education and Training Advisory Board (DTETAB) represented Dental Technicians. The Dental Technicians Association (DTA) was launched on 9 October 2002. This is not just a re-naming but a radical change in its image, concept and function. Building on the heritage of DTETAB in training and education, the DTA's role is to help prepare dental technicians in the build-up to statutory registration. The DTA has launched an internet site for easy access by members, together with a revamped newsletter. Coming shortly will be a free legal helpline, indemnity insurance and discount schemes. Their website can be found at www.dta-uk.org.

Section 2
Front-of-house Skills

Chapter 3
Front-of-house Communication

Communicating with colleagues

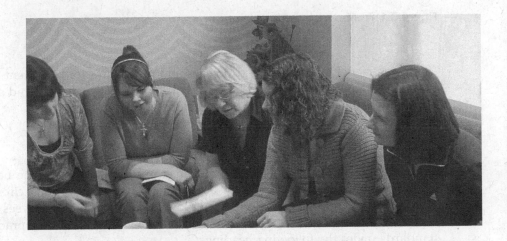

In workplaces throughout the world, lifelong friendships are formed between co-workers; dental practices are no exception. Many dental professionals describe the nature of their team as 'family like'. These close personal and professional relationships can create supportive and nurturing teams, although it is important to note that when relationships fail the consequences can be devastating, as in the break-up of a family. Since a close-knit community can result from good interpersonal relationships within a team, it is vital to recognise the importance of establishing excellent communications to bond the practice community.

Effective communication calls upon a wide range of innate and learned skills and requires the active co-operation of individuals and the practice management team. The hub of practice communications is the reception; here the quality of communications will have a major impact upon business and interpersonal relationships. The communication role of reception is to form a link between all parts of the practice as shown in Figure 3.1.

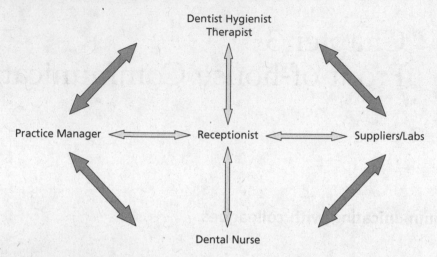

Figure 3.1 Front-desk communications.

For this model to work, agreed policies and procedures for consistent and effective communication should be recorded in the practice manual and supported by willingness among team members.

Practice manual

The introduction of a practice manual brings numerous benefits, one being the clarification of expectations by outlining what, under various circumstances, the practice requires from its employees and what the employees can expect from the practice. A typical practice manual will communicate practice standards under the following headings:

Company structure
Organisational chart.

Personnel management
(1)   Statement of employment.
(2)   Mission statement.
(3)   Service standards.
(4)   Practice rules.
(5)   Team development.
(6)   Team meetings.
(7)   Inductions.
(8)   Appraisals.
(9)   Communication.
(10)   Disciplinary – grievance procedures.
(11)   Medical treatment.

(12) Confidentiality rules.
(13) Equal opportunities.
(14) Substance abuse policy.
(15) Anti-discrimination or harassment policy.
(16) Fire regulations.

Practice development

(1)   Communications with head office.
(2)   Computer usage.
(3)   Data protection.
(4)   Freedom of Information Act.
(5)   Telephone protocols.
(6)   Patients' rights.
(7)   Administrative systems.
(8)   Monitoring systems.
(9)   Infection control.
(10) Health and safety.
(11) Marketing.
(12) Patients' terms and conditions.
(13) Complaints procedure.
(14) Practice information leaflet.

When expectations are clarified and well communicated, they become the foundation of a fair and equitable workplace environment.

> Many practices have a practice manual in some form. Unfortunately it often sits unused on a remote shelf. Ideally the practice manual is a multi-purpose tool for new and established team members, providing information and working instructions. Therefore, it must always be up to date and accessible to everyone. Some practices give each team member their own printed version. This can, however, be expensive because of its size. Worse still, complications arise when updates are made, as you have to rely on people replacing the old pages in their manual with the updated pages provided.
>
> Now that computer technology is well established in many practices, it is advisable to print a master copy of the manual, and then give each team member their copy burned on to a CD. Better still, when practices are planning their websites, if they choose a format with a team-only section the manual can be made available to the team through the practice website.

Standardising working instructions

The creation of your manual should be a team project, with each person contributing working instructions and standards for their job description. Once agreed and written down, these become a training manual for new team members. In this way, when inducting new staff, first-generation instructions are readily available for work tasks rather than instructions diluted by the Chinese whispers syndrome. When writing the manual pages for their job description, team members will give thought to the way they work. This can lead to the discovery of more efficient and effective ways of working.

With clarified expectations setting the scene for effective communication between colleagues, it is possible to build a comfort zone based on routines, empathy and respect. To cultivate this kind of environment, with each member of the team playing their part, communications need to be focused and have:

- a transparent and common purpose (possibly not stated but understood);
- agreed channels such as memos, Win-pops, notes, the spoken word, etc.

With these communication basics in place, the success of the communication will depend upon co-operation between the parties in the following ways:

- Both parties must want to communicate.
- Both parties should be prepared to see the other's point of view.
- Written communications must be appropriate, clear and concise.
- Skilled techniques should be applied to telephone communications.

The importance of both parties participating in the communication process cannot be understated. When the results of communications are disappointing, it is important to identify where the process can be strengthened to improve future results. Communication chain theory offers just this opportunity.

The communication chain

In social and workplace situations communication is the most important skill. Where respectful and consistent communication channels are in place, there is a greater likelihood that harmonious and respectful relationships will be formed. When communications are erratic or disrespectful, the impact upon the whole practice will be detrimental and far reaching. The management must set the rules and channels for communication and the team must understand and follow those rules. As with all management activities, research, design, planning and implementation of communication processes are essential to ensure the best possible chance of success.

Effective communication results when messages are sent, received and understood. Problems caused by poor communication can severely undermine motivation, reputations and credibility. For some people, communicating comes as naturally as breathing, whereas for others it calls for

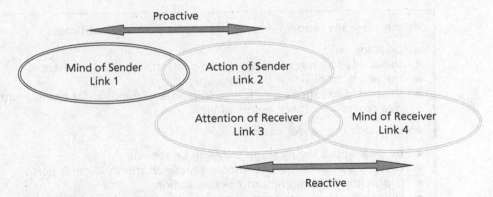

Figure 3.2 The communication chain.

considerable effort, requiring them to muster every possible ounce of courage to overcome their introversions. When workplace communications or inhibitions rely wholly on individuals' aptitudes and emotional responses, there will be inconsistencies leading to conflict. To ensure consistently successful communications, an understanding of the communication process is required; this process is aptly defined using the analogy of the communication chain. In the same way that a chain is only as strong as its weakest link, the communication process is a series of interlinked processes, integrated to allow messages to pass from the sender to the receiver for interpretation.

The communication chain, as shown in Figure 3.2, is a four-stage process, recognising the two-way nature of communication. This framework allows the identification of the results of actions and responses at the links of the chain, enabling us to evaluate and develop skills and leading to improved communications.

The first two links of the communication chain involve activities from the *sender*. These are the proactive stages of communication, which lead on to the reactive activities of the *receiver*, through whom messages are received and interpreted. Having interpreted the message, the receiver may well choose to become the sender of a response, requiring activities from links 1 and 2 of the communication chain.

Link 1 of the communication chain: the mind of the sender

At this stage of the communication chain the essential thinking processes that precede action take place. At link 1, the need to communicate is recognised and the sender decides what they want from the communication. The sender needs to begin an initial research process. On occasion this will be a formal information-gathering process involving considerable amounts of time and resources, whilst at other times it will be a simple process of following an agreed protocol.

At this stage the sender needs the following skills and aptitudes:

- planning skills;
- the ability to express emotions and deal with emotional others;
- the ability to deliver a clear message;
- the ability to express a differing opinion and stand up for oneself with due regard for others' points of view.

At this stage the sender needs to:

- be clear about the message they will be sending;
- decide upon the action or response required from the other person;
- choose the right method of communication;
- choose the right language.

Link 2 of the communication chain: the action of the sender

Here the sender acts upon the thinking from link 1. When actions at this link are consistent with the identified outcomes, the chances of effective communication are reinforced and the communication process moves on to link 3, the attention of the receiver. However, if the act is incoherent or badly implemented, the communication chain will break and the possibility of a successful outcome will be lost.

In terms of the written communication at link 2 of the communication chain, memos, notes, reports and notices, used appropriately and assertively, provide good communication channels.

The skills and aptitudes required for success at link 2 of the chain are:

- the ability to open a conversation;
- writing skills;
- the ability to read others;
- the ability to give constructive criticism;
- empathy;
- diplomacy;
- assertiveness;
- the ability to choose the right language.

It is vital to choose a suitable time and place for the communication. These choices will be made at link 1 and enacted at link 2. Finding the right time and place requires empathy, diplomacy and assertiveness. At this stage the sender needs to:

- *Choose the right communication medium*: 80% of communication is non-verbal, delivered through body language, social perception and timing. It is not so much what you say as the way that you say it. We deliver non-verbal signals through posture, gestures, facial expression and voice.
- *Be assertive*: Assertiveness is a widely misunderstood concept. Look at the following behavioural characteristics of being assertive, non-assertive and aggressive:

- To be *non-assertive* is to fail to stand up for yourself effectively, often handing over responsibility for your well-being to another person.
- To be *aggressive* is to violate the rights of others. Aggressive behaviour is not always straightforward. People who behave in apparently passive ways can nevertheless violate the rights of others through manipulation, non-cooperation, or dumb insolence.
- To be *assertive* is to stand up for yourself and your rights while not violating the rights of others in the process. You will listen rather than defend, question rather than grudgingly accept.

■ *Choose the right time and place*: Choosing the right time to have a word with a colleague is critically important. For example waiting to have a 'private word' about something that concerns you would have a different impact from speaking out in a group or public place. Neither approach is wholly right or wrong, simply a matter of choice, following decisions made at link 1 of the chain.

Link 3 of the communication chain: the attention of the receiver

Communication cannot be achieved unless both parties are active in the communication process. Before a message can be interpreted, it must be received. *This stage of the chain is purely sensory.* Unless the message is brought to the attention of the receiver, the communication process cannot be completed.

Only when the communication has been brought to the attention of the receiver can the communication process proceed. If you wrote a letter but forgot to post it, the information it contains could not reach the receiver's attention so the communication would fail. In the same way as if a letter arrives for you and you choose not to read it, so too, when a receiver does not listen to a sender's verbal message, communication breaks down.

Listening is a vital communication activity

There are three things to remember about listening:

■ *Listening and hearing are not the same*: Hearing is only one stage of the complex process of listening. Hearing is the physical act of receiving sounds. This could be expressed in another way:
■ *You hear with your ears, but you listen with your mind.*
■ *Listening does not just happen*: Listening requires mental energy, unflagging attention and an effort to understand. When you listen with concentration, the following physical changes occur.

  - Pulse quickens.
  - Body temperature rises.
  - Pupils of the eyes dilate.

To fully understand how being listened to enhances communication, try the listening exercise outlined in Figure 3.3.

Listening exercise

For this exercise you will need the help of two colleagues; ask one person to be the 'sender' and one the 'receiver'.

Stage 1
(1) Ask the sender to tell the listener five things they do for pleasure and relaxation.
(2) Ask the receiver to give no visual or verbal signs that they are listening to the sender.

Observe the body language of both parties.

Stage 2
(1) Ask the sender and receiver to switch roles and replay stage 1 above.
(2) Ask the sender to describe how they felt during the exercise about:

  ■ their chosen activities;
  ■ how they were treated by their 'receiver'.

Stage 3
(1) Now ask the sender to identify something they would like to put into 'Room 101'. This will be a trivial irritation that they would like to get rid of. Ask them to tell the receiver what this would be and why it irritates them.
(2) This time ask the receiver to give their full attention to the receiver, mirroring their body language, giving eye contact and smiling as appropriate.

Stage 4
Ask the sender and receiver to switch roles and replay stage 3.

Discuss with the participants how they experienced both types of listening.

Figure 3.3 Listening exercise.

Listening is a grossly underestimated and immensely powerful tool of communication. At this stage both the sender and receiver are participating in the communication, i.e. you speak, whilst I listen.

The skills and aptitudes required for success at link 3 of the communication chain are:

■ active listening;
■ rapport building skills;
■ checking the meaning of the message if you are unsure;
■ provide feedback to show your understanding;
■ give the sender the chance to amend the message.

Listening is a learned behaviour that can be improved. Once the message has been received, the process of interpretation begins, leading on to the fourth and final stage of the communication chain.

Link 4 of the communication chain: mind of the receiver

We each view the world around us in our own individual way. Psychologist George Kelly believes we see the world through the light of our past experiences and in this way we form a personalised knowledge of the world and expectations of how it should be. We use these constructs to make value judgements, based upon our attitudes, values and beliefs. At times, these judgements lead us to resist, reject or ignore certain communications. Even if the sender's part in communication has been carried out perfectly well, the receiver may choose to block or reject the message. It is only when all stages of the chain have been completed successfully that the communication process is complete.

> The skills and aptitudes required for success at link 4 of the communication chain are:
>
> ■ confidence and friendliness;
> ■ perception of others' feelings;
> ■ empathy;
> ■ respect for others.

When the communication has reached this stage of the chain it is possible to evaluate the extent to which it has achieved its objectives. The value of the communication chain is that it provides a method of examining activities at each stage to assess where skills need further development.

Barriers to communication at link 4 of the communication chain

Inattentive listening
Difficulties in paying attention can be due to psychological or environmental factors, or to a lack of interest in what the sender is saying. It may well be that the sender is using language that the receiver cannot identify with or understand. In many cases the receiver's feeling about the sender or the potential benefits of the message will influence the amount of effort devoted to listening.

Interrupting whilst others speak
Cutting people off, finishing their sentences or jumping in with your own opinions can be tempting if you feel the sender is taking too long with the communication. This can be due to the receiver's state of mind and the pressures they are working under. As a sender you need to be perceptive of the receiver's state of mind and as a receiver you need to be aware of your habit and re-train yourself.

Defensiveness
When we regard people with differing points of view as a threat, we become defensive. At times we are right to be aware of the personal safety issues linked to aggression from others. However, this is rarely likely to be an

imminent danger. Try not to take differences personally: look at them as opportunities to broaden your understanding of others.

Offensive criticism

If you are making a complaint, try not to use language and techniques that put others on the defensive. Always focus on the behaviour rather than the person you have the issue with, and do not resort to name calling or making wild generalisations. Keep a calm, even tone of voice and ensure you have relaxed body language.

Lack of emotional control

When communications are emotionally charged, it can be difficult to remain calm. Try to pick the time and place to deal with such issues. Learn some calming methods and ensure that you gather your thoughts before dealing with touchy subjects.

Conflict avoidance

When you know that the communication you need to deliver may upset the receiver, you could be tempted to put it off or dilute the message, sometimes to the extent that it becomes unable to achieve its objectives. Take time to plan and prepare, and make sure you deliver the message. Speak sensitively and assertively.

When you communicate you use your whole body and mind, not just your words. As a sender, plan your communications with the listener in mind. As a receiver, develop listening and rapport-building skills. Be alert and aware, and improve your communication skills through practice and evaluation. Communication skills are the lifeblood of any workplace; effective communications are the basis of healthy, respectful, interpersonal relationships between colleagues, leading to happy, productive and cooperative teams.

Communicating with patients

Everyone in the team has a role to play in communication with patients. The British Dental Receptionists' Association considered the receptionist's role in patient communications to be so important that they entitled their inaugural Annual Conference, 'First Impressions', to reflect their belief that receptionists are 'managing directors of first impressions'.

Patients do not visit the practice to see the receptionist. However, research carried out by the BDRA indicates that patients unhappy with the receptionist's attitude are less likely to return to the practice than those unhappy with the dentist's attitude. This may be because many patients do not expect pleasant experiences in the treatment room, but expect to be treated with courtesy and respect in reception, comparing their experiences at the practice with their customer care experiences from retail, service and financial services sectors. Dental practices therefore need to develop customer care measures built upon the values of these sectors, with which we are in direct competition for patients' disposable income.

Reception teams need to develop clear, courteous systems and services that patients will experience as respectful and caring. Well planned, consistent customer-care systems lead to co-operative relationships. This can only be achieved through communication channels which are planned, recorded (in a procedures manual) and communicated to staff.

The managing director of first impressions
Creating the right impression

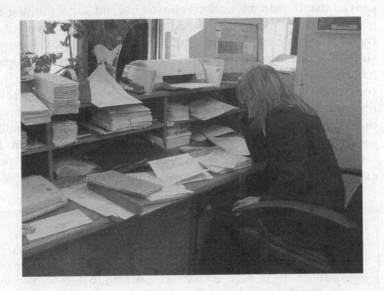

Over time we become so accustomed to our everyday workplace surroundings that we become oblivious to the first impressions given to patients entering the practice for the first time. Interestingly, when practices conduct patient satisfaction surveys, they regularly collect unexpected feedback on the layout or colour scheme in the reception area. This shows how important the reception and waiting areas are to patients. The comfort and quality of these areas convey the practice's attitude to patient comfort.

Research shows that, for many patients, the time spent in the waiting room is the most anxious part of their visit to the dentist – particularly when they can hear the sounds from the treatment room, such as drills and suction! So it's important to make the waiting room as calm and pleasant as possible. An airy and uncluttered reception area can add to a sense of calm.

When coupled with efficient and considerate customer care procedures, patients' anxieties can be considerably reduced.

Always leave the reception area tidy at the end of the day, ready for the next morning. It will be one thing less to organise at the start of the next busy day. Your reception area may include a waiting area. If so, check that the magazines, comics, books and toys are in good condition. Check your displays and restock as required.

Greeting patients at reception

Verbal communication plays a crucial part in human relationships. When two people first meet each other, perceptions formed at that time form the basis of their relationship. During the 1950s, psychologist Eric Berne studied people's interactions and formed his theories of transactional analysis which to this day are widely used to predict and explain human relationships. Berne's research proved that human interactions go well beyond social training and good manners; they are an intrinsic part of our personality and essential to our well-being. By making eye contact, smiling and speaking politely, we are giving 'positive strokes' which increase comfort and co-operation between people. On the other hand, by failing to recognise the presence of another person, not making eye contact or using terse language, you deliver a negative stroke, a powerful rejection, leading the other person to feel affronted and either react with anger, or withdraw from the interaction. Negative strokes have a spiralling effect, with each reaction being a response to a previous negative reaction. Therefore, procedures for greeting patients as they arrive should feature positive strokes, even when the receptionist is working under pressure in a busy reception.

Such a procedure would include the following measures:

(1) *Acknowledge the presence of the patient with eye contact and a smile within five seconds of their arrival*. Eye contact can be made with the patient at the desk, even when speaking to another patient in person or over the telephone. This is not an unreasonable requirement of the receptionist, and it delivers a powerful positive stroke, especially when supported by a smile.

(2) *Whenever possible address patients using their name*. Using a person's name shows that you recognise them as a person, rather than just 'the next patient'.

(3) *Open the dialogue with an appropriate version of 'Hello'*. The most appropriate version of 'Hello' will depend upon how well you know the patient and local social norms. This greeting is simple good manners, and shows respect to the patient rather than launching into conversation without due recognition of the person to whom you are speaking.

(4) *Ask the patient to take a seat and inform them of any delays likely to affect their appointment*. Keeping patients advised of delays can reduce their anxiety and give them the option to rearrange their appointment if the delay is so long as to be unacceptable to them. Otherwise you can enable them to use the time they would have spent in your waiting room elsewhere, e.g. visiting a local shop or taking a walk.

Persuasion and Negotiation

Much of your time at work is spent negotiating with patients, colleagues, representatives or official bodies. At times you will need to use skills of persuasion to change the other person's point of view. This can be difficult. However, if you handle the situation well, you can influence the outcome. Negotiating involves transferring facts, ideas, attitudes or opinions from one person to another in order to change a point of view.

Q: How can you persuade someone to take a different course of action from the one that they have decided upon?

A: By presenting a case that is irrefutable, constructed in a way that provokes thought and earns respect.

(1)   First, think things through and clarify what you want the outcome to be.

(2)   Identify what outcome the other person wants. Anticipate their responses and prepare your answers to points they will raise.

(3)   Make sure that your ideas are realistic and presented in terms that the other person can relate to.

(4)   Present your ideas so that the other person can change their point of view without losing face.

(5)   Give factual evidence; do not exaggerate or minimise.

These are vital skills for receptionists as mediators between patients and the dental team, and between the team and the public. What makes one person more persuasive than another? Psychologists believe that the key factor may be an ability to inspire trust. A trusting person feels more relaxed. Once trust has been established, patients feel more relaxed.

Keeping up appearances

A well groomed, smart, clean and tidy receptionist projects a professional image. Hair and hands are particularly important; make sure both are clean and tidy. Try to see yourself through the patient's eyes: to see yourself as they see you when entering the practice.

An area of considerable debate is whether or not receptionists should wear nurses' uniforms. As uniforms communicate to patients who we are and what we do, we should consider the intrinsic messages in what we wear and not send misleading messages.

Name badges can be a friendly and efficient way of personalising the team to patients. Care should be taken to minimise the possibility of nuisance contacts from patients outside of work hours by only showing first names and job roles on badges.

Practice information leaflets (PILs)

Since the early 1990s practice information leaflets have been used by smart practices to communicate services and terms of business to patients. Websites are increasingly replacing or supplementing the information provided by PILs.

Freedom of Information Act

On 1 January 2005 the Freedom of Information Act became law, giving the public a right to certain information about public services including dental practices. As small businesses, practices need to be aware that the Act includes obligations for certain information such as business plans and pricing policies to be made public. With this in mind, it makes good business sense to make this information readily available in a format that gives patients all the information they need to make informed choices about their dental care. This willingness to share information also helps promote the practice.

Another form of legal compliance you can address is to confirm the arrangements you have made under the Disability Rights Act. From 1 October 2004, dental practices must show they have taken all reasonable measures to make their services accessible to patients with disabilities. You need to highlight any facilities such as wheelchair access, hearing loops, etc. In addition to the practice owner's responsibilities under the terms of this Act, receptionists also have a responsibility towards patients, ensuring they do everything possible to help patients with disabilities to access services.

When visiting a practice for the first time, some patients may have difficulty locating it or finding a parking place. When researching why new patients failed their first appointments, practices have often found that they could not find a parking place and returned home rather than be late. Practices that cannot make parking available can warn patients and help them by providing a list of local car parks. Details of local bus services and bus stops are also helpful to patients visiting for the first time.

Written communications

Computers play a major role in dental practice administration. Some previously handwritten letters can be typed and stored electronically. Senior team members develop these letters for ease of use and reception staff personalise copies for patients as required. It is vitally important to review them regularly to ensure they are current and appropriate. Written communications in this category include:

- recall reminders;
- accounts;
- failed appointment follow-ups;

- cancellation letters;
- referral letters;
- treatment plans and estimates.

Lab sheets

Some handwritten communications, such as entering correct dates on to lab sheets, are essential to the smooth running of treatment rooms. Policies must be in place to ensure that such written communications are carried out to a satisfactory standard and achieve consistent results.

Treatment plans and estimates

Dento-legal requirements specify that patients must be given full and detailed explanations of treatment plans and cost estimates. However, experience shows that no matter how much time and effort are spent in the treatment room explaining treatment details, anxious patients frequently seek reassurance from the receptionist about their treatment; this often reflects patients' perceived lack of knowledge and understanding of dental procedures. Before our explanations can enable patients to make informed choices, we need to enable them to understand their care options by ensuring as far as possible that our explanations are jargon free.

Mind your language

Jargon is a useful form of shorthand used between colleagues with a shared understanding of its meaning. To outsiders, however, it is meaningless and can lead to feelings of inadequacy. Figure 3.4 outlines the response I was given in a computer retail shop when I asked about a computer. Although it was no doubt technically correct, it left me no wiser about the computer in question so I had to ask my companion what it all meant.

Because receptionists are more likely to use lay terms in their explanations, patients turn to them for guidance. It is therefore essential that receptionists are fully aware of what their dentists will have already said to the patient, in order to ensure that they are reinforcing their messages rather than contradicting them.

This computer has two processors running at 2.5 GHz, which are capable of symmetric multiprocessing.

It has 1 gigabyte of PC3200 error correction code, random access memory and a RAID 5 fault-tolerant volume attached to an ultra-wide SCSI adaptor.

Figure 3.4 Jargon.

Telephone skills

The majority of first contacts that patients make with the practice are over the telephone. Because of the importance of first impressions, developing good telephone skills is very important. The style in which the telephone is answered in your practice should be set out in practice policy. In this way a standardised telephone technique will project a consistent professionalism in customer care.

A matter of heated debate in many practices is whether a ringing telephone should take precedence over the patient at the desk. In many cases practice protocols state that the phone should be answered within five rings, so receptionists excuse themselves from patients at the desk and answer the phone. Most patients are fine with this if it happens occasionally. When it happens several times during one conversation, it delivers a negative stroke leading to irritation. If the patient has time pressures, it can lead to a formal complaint.

Now that many practices use computerised appointment systems, there is no longer a need for the appointment book to be sited on the front desk. This gives practices the freedom to move the telephones from the front desk into a back office. In this way the role of receptionist on the front desk is one of care coordinator taking care of 'patient present' activities, with a colleague in a back office taking care of the telephones.

Clear protocols for answering the telephone should be communicated to anyone answering the practice phone. There is no universal code for this. The right protocols for your practice will create an impression of professionalism to the caller, whilst feeling natural and comfortable to the receptionist delivering them.

The greeting should be clear and concise. Long detailed greetings are lost on callers, who usually respond by saying 'Is that the dentist's?'. Most receptionists find that something as simple as 'Hello, Family Dental Care. How can I help you?' delivered in a well moderated tone will open the conversation most effectively.

When developing your practice's telephone answering protocols it is worth while considering the points shown in Figure 3.5. Please make use of the grid to identify aspects of your practice's telephone protocols.

Most receptionists will tell you that the most rewarding part of their work is patient contact. The dental profession as a whole is becoming increasingly aware of the importance of good interpersonal skills for building mutually rewarding relationships. The foundations of good relationships are respectful communications, which are much too important to be left to luck. Clearly defined and agreed protocols are the essence of good communications.

Customer care need	Protocol
Be aware of how the phone is answered and that it impacts on the patient's image of the practice.	Our standard response for answering the phone is........................
Remember that patients like to be addressed by name.	Write down caller's name as a matter of routine at the beginning of a call, and refer to the caller by name during the call.
A friendly response.	Put a smile in your voice, by smiling when talking on the phone.
Give the caller your undivided attention.	Never carry on a conversation with someone else when you are talking on the phone. Never eat or drink when taking a call.
A method of contacting the practice 24 hours a day.	Use the answering machine when you are too busy to respond to telephone calls.
A professional response.	When placing callers on hold, use the 'privacy' button. Double-check that the patient has understood what you have said to them. Close conversations polite and courteously.

Figure 3.5 Creating telephone protocols.

Communicating with suppliers

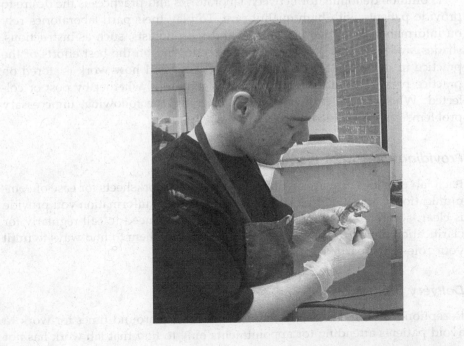

Dental businesses are successful when they meet the needs of both their internal and external customers. External customers are the patients who purchase goods and services, whereas internal customers are people who enable the practice to trade, by providing goods and services. This group includes the dental team and suppliers of goods and services.

The importance of communicating effectively with colleagues and patients is understood. However, other groups vital to the smooth running of the practice are frequently overlooked, namely laboratories and dental representatives, who should be regarded as part of the team and considered when setting procedures or protocols that affect them. Because contact made with these groups is generally at arm's length, over the phone, by e-mail or by post, it is especially important to create effective communication channels designed to enable them to identify and meet your requirements.

Mutually respectful relationships between practices and dental laboratories result when both parties invest in relationship building, communicating their needs and expectations of each other. Where laboratories are situated on practice premises, everyone benefits from day-to-day contact as technicians become an integral part of the team. When working with external laboratories, it is especially important to nurture cooperative relationships.

Many of the restrictions and challenges of running a profitable practice are mirrored in dental laboratories, and just like dental practices they need to inform and educate customers to build good relationships. Forward-thinking laboratories invest time and energy in developing rapport with dentists, nurses and receptionists. Some have training rooms on their premises and invite practice groups to 'getting to know you' meetings.

A common denominator between laboratories and practices is the desire to provide patients with high quality care. To play their part, laboratories rely on information from dentists, nurses and receptionists, such as instructions, shades, and 'required by' dates. They also depend on the best efforts of the practice in respect of the quality of impressions and how work is stored on practice premises and transported to the laboratory, whether by post or collected. When agreed protocols are in place for the following, unnecessary problems can be avoided.

Providing clear work instructions

Each lab provides practices with their specialised worksheets for ease of communication. Care should be taken to ensure that the information you provide is clear, accurate and sufficient. If your technicians need to call regularly for clarification of instructions, you need to work with them to find ways to fulfil your role in the partnership.

Delivery procedures

Reception staff must be aware of delivery and turnaround times for work to avoid patients attending for appointments only to find that lab work has not been returned. Wise receptionists build in a 'time cushion' so that errors can be rectified before the patient arrives. It is advisable for the receptionist to have a checklist of the work expected in each delivery.

When work is posted to labs, great care should be taken to ensure that the packaging is sufficiently protective, that all instructions are included in the package, that the lab's address is clearly shown on the front of the package and the practice address is also shown (as the sender) on the back of the package, and that the correct amount of postage is purchased.

When a lab representative calls to collect work, make sure that you are ready for their visit, with all work to be transported gathered in the correct place and 'return by dates' clearly shown on lab sheets.

Cross-infection control

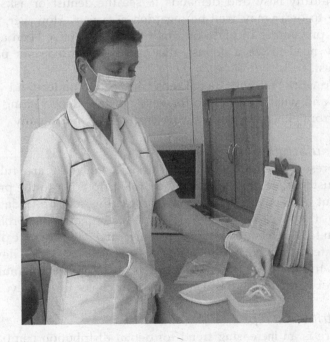

Lab work will be exposed to saliva, and at times to mixtures of blood and saliva, from patients' mouths, which may be contaminated with a wide variety of microorganisms including blood-borne viruses. Patients carrying blood-borne viruses may be asymptomatic and unaware of their infectious status. In the absence of screening of all patients for known infections, all blood and saliva must be considered infectious. It is essential that cross-infection procedures be followed before work is forwarded to labs since the potential for transferring infections is well documented. Pathogens are transferred to labs via impressions, appliances and dentures. Cross-infection measures will be dependent upon the materials involved. New cross-infection products are introduced regularly to the dental market, and practices should develop and review their procedures.

Payments

In the same way that practices need patients to settle their accounts on time, labs are small businesses dependent on regular cash flow to survive. Many labs encounter difficulties when they have to wait for extended periods for payments. Careful records should be available in the practice to verify monthly statements, and payment should be made promptly.

Working with dental reps

A rep who arrives at the practice without notice when the practice is frantically busy and demands to see the dentist or asks what you would like to order may well be regarded as a pest. However, when the practice has procedures in place on times to call that have been agreed with reps if they need to see a dentist, they can be regarded as a partner rather than a pest.

To work best with dental reps you need to understand whom they represent and what they can do for your practice. Reps visiting your practice will be from either a manufacturing or distribution company.

Manufacturing reps

Representatives from manufacturing companies are fully trained dental industry professionals. Since their role is to bring to the practice information about innovative new products, procedures, and up-to-date quality information, they will ask to see the dentists. As marketing professionals they are keen to hear the 'voice of the customer' and will take note of customers' needs and feed them back to their designers to enable them to develop future products to fulfil these needs. Any orders you place with manufacturing reps will be forwarded to the distributor of your choice for supply.

Distribution reps

There is an increasing trend for dental distribution companies to deal with their customers over the internet rather than by sending reps from practice to practice. This enables them to be more competitive on price.

Irrespective of how you order practice consumables, it is important to have clear stock control procedures to ensure that you do not run out of materials. Stock control systems are most effective when someone has overall responsibility for their operation and a budget in order to ensure the most effective use of practice moneys.

Dental practices can become quite isolated, with little contact with other practices. Dental reps can provide a valuable grapevine. When the principles of effective teamwork are expanded to include everyone involved in making the practice work, the potential benefits are considerable. In most cases, dental suppliers are ready and willing to share their knowledge and expertise in areas of dentistry that may not necessarily exist within your team. By building mutually respectful and beneficial relationships with suppliers, you add skills to your team and value to your working experience.

Chapter 4
Understanding Patients' Rights

Confidentiality

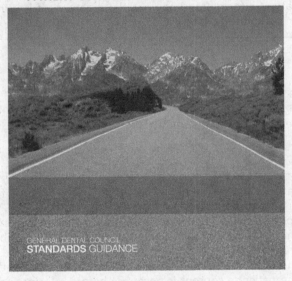

PRINCIPLES OF
PATIENT CONFIDENTIALITY

GENERAL DENTAL COUNCIL
STANDARDS GUIDANCE

As every receptionist knows, many patients are not exactly overjoyed to be visiting the dentist. With this in mind, it is important to develop sensitive and responsive reception services to ensure that every visit is as pleasant an experience as possible for the patient. Having a pleasing manner and giving a warm welcome to patients on arrival is the first step towards increasing patient comfort, although on their own such measures do not go far enough to provide the level of professionalism patients have a right to expect from their dental care providers.

The ethical guidance, *Standards for Dental Professionals*, published by the General Dental Council, sets the ethical principles that define professionalism in dentistry. Full and up-to-date details are readily available to the profession and patients on the GDC website, www.gdc-uk.org. The standards cover six key principles, each of which should be considered when creating reception working procedures. Although receptionists are not registered dental professionals in their own right, their employers are vicariously liable for their acts and omissions in respect of meeting standards set out in the GDC guidance.

Receptionists play an important role in ensuring that the practice maintains high ethical standards, particularly in respect of protecting patients' right to confidentiality. The GDC guidance, Principles for Confidentiality, says:

- Treat information about patients as confidential and only use it for the purposes for which it is given.
- Prevent information from being accidentally revealed and prevent unauthorised access by keeping information secure at all times.
- In exceptional circumstances, it may be justified to make confidential patient information known without consent if it is in the public interest or the patient's interest.

'Principles of Confidentiality' details rights and duties and clarifies circumstances under which information can be disclosed. Dental professionals must observe the following standards:

- Patients are entitled to expect that you will keep information about them confidential.
- Confidentiality is central to the trust between patient and dentist.
- The same duty of confidentiality applies to all members of the dental team.
- The right to confidentiality continues after a patient's death.
- The patient's consent is necessary before information is disclosed, and only the minimum information for the purpose must be given.

Every working day, receptionists encounter situations in which they could unintentionally disclose confidential information about patients. This could be when responding to an enquiry on the phone from an employer, school or relatives asking about a patient's whereabouts, or being overheard when talking to patients. Care should be taken to ensure receptionists are fully aware of practice policy on keeping information confidential, as patients could take legal action if they consider that their rights have been breached.

When other health professionals involved in the patient's care make requests for clinical information, the request must be forwarded to the patient's dentist or their clinical director who will decide how to respond. When making their decisions, they will keep in mind the need to justify their decisions and any action they take in the matter.

Data Protection Law requirements run in tandem with patient confidentiality requirements in respect of any non-clinical information held about patients. All patient information should be up to date, stored and disposed of with due regard to confidentiality.

> Receptionists should be aware that young people over the age of 16 are entitled to the same level of confidentiality as adult patients and information cannot be disclosed to their parents without their permission.

When designing the reception area, thought should be given to patients' need for privacy. It is essential to create an area in which patients can talk to the receptionist without being overheard. Many receptionists find it impossible to have private conversations with patients because the reception desk is the focal point of the waiting room and its activities attract attention. When possible, it is advisable to arrange seating in such a way that it is not directly facing and is at a respectful distance away from the reception desk. When dealing with a queue of patients at the reception desk, receptionists should insist that a courteous distance be maintained between the patient they are working with and the next person in the queue.

Every receptionist must be aware of how breaches of confidentiality can occur in routine work situations. The practice should provide training and guidance on how these can be avoided. In this way the receptionist faced with any situation in which a patient's rights could be breached should be able to refer to agreed protocols rather than having to make on-the-spot decisions.

With a clear understanding of the guiding principles of confidentiality, procedures can be agreed for those circumstances when it is deemed necessary to release information in the 'public interest'. This could be appropriate when a patient puts their own or others' health and safety at serious risk, or if you think that you have confidential information that could be used to prevent or detect a serious crime, e.g. child abuse.

The trust between patients and their dental care providers is an essential part of their dental experience. Respectful reception services set the tone; the GDC standards are a valuable guide to how to organise services that will enhance patients' dental experiences.

Informed consent to treatment

PRINCIPLES OF
PATIENT CONSENT

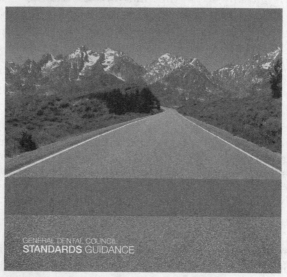

GENERAL DENTAL COUNCIL
STANDARDS GUIDANCE

The importance of the bond of trust between patients and their dentists should never be underestimated. Trust must be the cornerstone of the professional relationship and needs to be earned. Since most patients understand little of what happens to them in the dental chair, we must work to ensure they feel confident that their dentist is putting their needs first and acting in their best interests. When deciding whether to place their trust in a dental care provider, patients look to the aspects of their care they understand to justify their decisions.

> The esteem and dignity with which patients are treated by every member of the dental team will help to build trust and confidence. When patients feel they have been given the information required to make informed decisions about their dental care, the bond of trust is reinforced and more importantly patients can really appreciate the value rather than cost of their care.

Obtaining consent before examining a patient or starting treatment is an observation of their right to decide what happens to their body. This is a right that we must uphold, as failure to do so can lead to legal action. Dental professionals are required to work within the standards set by the

GDC, covering six main principles to safeguard patients' rights including principles of patient consent. The GDC publishes booklets providing details and guidance on the standards it expects, including specific guidance on Principles of Patient Consent. These can be downloaded from their website at www.gdc-uk.org.

> All clinicians should be well aware of the importance of ensuring every patient gives their consent to be treated after receiving a written treatment plan and cost estimate before starting their treatment. Patient's consent must be:
>
> **Informed**:   they must have enough information, in a format they can understand, to make a decision after weighing up the costs and benefits of the treatments offered. This is not a one-off process; it should be part of ongoing discussions with patients.
>
> **Voluntary**:   the decision to go ahead with treatment must be made by the patient.
>
> **Competent**:   patients must be able to make an informed decision.

Dentists can spend a great deal of time talking to patients and explaining treatment options, only to find they leave the treatment room and ask the receptionist questions about their treatment plan. Therefore, it is important that receptionists have a thorough understanding of procedures and treatments, how they are carried out and any risks attached to them. It is also essential that receptionists reinforce rather than contradict information given in the treatment room. This requires that receptionists be thoroughly briefed on how to respond to patients. It is essential that receptionists fully understand the concept of informed consent, so that they can underpin the work of the practice in ensuring that valid patient consent is always secured.

Besides clinical aspects of treatment, patients must be fully aware of the nature of the contract under which treatment is offered, and, in particular, whether they have been accepted for treatment under an NHS or private contract. In the beginning they must agree to the cost of the initial consultation and be given the probable cost of further treatments in a written treatment plan. If there are any changes to the original treatment plan, you must get the patient's consent to pay any additional costs, and provide an amended treatment plan.

Where barriers to communication exist, such as when patients have hearing or language difficulties, you must take reasonable steps to ensure that they can make an informed decision. This could be achieved by asking the patient to bring an interpreter with them, or by providing hearing loops.

Patients have a right to refuse or give partial consent for treatment. If they do so, this must be respected. Make sure you keep clear records and keep clinicians fully informed of any conversations you have with patients, during which they express concerns or reservations about treatment options.

Trust, consent to treatment and respect are interdependent facets of our relationships with patients, which every member of the team plays a role in building. To do so we must treat patients politely and with respect, in recognition of their dignity and rights as individuals.

Permitted duties

To protect the public from clinical incompetence, the Dentists Act limits 'the practice of dentistry' to qualified and registered practitioners. It is therefore illegal for a person who is not a registered dental professional to practise dentistry, or to lead others to believe they are practising or are prepared to practise dentistry.

> The Dentists Act of 1984 defines an act of dentistry as 'any such treatment, advice or attendance as is usually performed or given by dentists'. The Act specifies that acts of dentistry 'include the provision of any treatment and advice, in connection with the fitting, insertion or fixing of dentures or other dental appliances'.

Hygienists and therapists are currently permitted to perform specified duties. However, changes to the Dentists Act in 2006 allowed registrants of the GDC to practise dentistry within the limits of their training and competence. Registration was expanded to include not only dentists, hygienists and therapists, but also dental nurses, dental technicians, clinical dental technicians and orthodontic therapists. The GDC's publication *Developing the Dental Team* sets out the curricular frameworks for each of these groups. These define the duties in which each group will be expected to be competent.

Under the new legislation, the dentist undertakes an initial review of a patient and provides a treatment plan, the details of which will vary according to the patient's needs. For a patient with no significant oral health problems, the plan might be limited to specifying routine dental care and a reassessment interval of two to three years. The patient would be allowed to take this plan to any dental care registrant, who would be permitted, within the limits of the plan and of their training and competence, to provide any treatment and make any necessary referrals until the reassessment date. Patients with no teeth are allowed to see a clinical dental technician without prior review by a dentist.

As it is unlawful for an unregistered person to give or suggest they are prepared to give any advice on treatments, reception staff must ensure that they do not offer implicit or explicit advice to patients. However, where information has originated from a dental registrant and is written down in practice policy as the appropriate way to respond to specific queries, receptionists and practice managers can in certain cases act as a mediator between a registered clinician and the patient.

Clinical Governance

The dental profession enjoys the privilege of self-governing status. Maintaining this status is wholly dependent upon maintaining the confidence of the population. To achieve this, the profession must be seen to be consistently acting in patient's best interests.

The Clinical Governance initiative was introduced in 2001 to provide evidence of the profession's highest intentions, sincerest efforts and commitment to excellence in the provision of dental care. Under Clinical Governance regulations, practices are required to produce evidence of the implementation of well defined and recorded management systems. Clinical Governance measures are part of the terms of service for providers of NHS dentistry.

Clinical Governance is not limited to dental care providers. It is a Department of Health initiative applying to all sectors of the National Health Service and is defined by the Department of Health as

'A system through which NHS organisations are accountable for continuously improving the quality of their services and safeguarding high standards of care by creating an environment in which excellence in clinical care will flourish.'

To meet this standard, practices must provide evidence of having set benchmark standards, recorded performance to standard and evaluated results to establish best practice for:

- risk management;
- evidence-based dentistry;
- quality indicators;
- handling patient feedback;
- learning from experience;
- measuring performance;
- professional development;
- sharing ideas.

Responsibility and accountability

With the modernisation of NHS dentistry under the Options for Change Initiative, the Primary Care Trusts (PCTs) became responsible for monitoring Clinical Governance compliance. Guidelines are provided in the Clinical Governance Kit of the British Dental Association (BDA).

BDA Clinical Governance Kit

The BDA Clinical Governance Kit supports practices in the implementation of their Clinical Governance measures and strongly advocates the production of a practice manual to set benchmarks and service standards and maintain consistency in services.

> The materials in the Kit are compiled to take practices step by step towards the development of measures to address the following nine components of Clinical Governance:
>
> - the patient experience;
> - patient, carer, service user and public involvement;
> - clinical effectiveness;
> - risk management;
> - education, training and continuous professional development;
> - use of information;
> - clinical audit;
> - staffing and staff management;
> - strategic capacity (implementation of Clinical Governance).

For Clinical Governance measures to realise their full potential requires an inclusive team approach. Teams need to define roles and responsibilities to meet each of the nine components.

Receptionists in particular have frequent opportunities to observe patients and to give feedback to the team during team meetings on patients' comments, compliments and complaints. Some medical practices actually appoint patient representatives, who attend their planning meetings to ensure patients' perspectives are considered when making decisions about services.

Measuring the effectiveness of clinical care is usually the responsibility of clinicians, in particular clinical directors. However, the reception team can play a role by gathering data from the appointment book, for example on waiting times, lost fillings or denture eases, to produce valuable comparative information for each clinician.

Under the Management of Health and Safety at Work Regulations 1999, in any workplace where four or more people are employed, risk assessments must be conducted and recorded. Full details of risk assessment requirements are outlined in Chapter 12 of this book which covers planning and management systems.

The concept of lifelong learning and the ongoing development of technical skills are central to all professions, with their regulatory bodies (in the case of dentistry the GDC) requiring evidence of practitioners' continuous professional development (CPD) as a condition of continued registration. In some professions, CPD has been expanded to CPPD, continuous professional and personal development, showing the importance of a holistic approach to ongoing development. The GDC sets the standards for CPD for dental professionals; many willingly exceed the prescribed hours, regarding their professional development as an essential and enjoyable aspect of their professional life. Many choose to spread their learning between clinical, management and interpersonal skills to enhance patient services and team relationships.

Good communications are the core of Clinical Governance. They necessitate the sharing of information with other professionals through peer review groups, which promotes the dissemination of knowledge. Practice meetings should be held frequently in ring-fenced time, and an accurate account of proceedings must be kept in the meeting minutes.

The ability to conduct audit processes, collating factual information for comparison of results to target, is an essential skill for quality management. Here dental care professionals can support their clinicians by collecting some of the raw data required for clinical audit.

It has become increasingly clear over the past 10 years that practice management should feature more prominently in undergraduate and vocational dental training. Before quality of care can be central to practices' values, those values must extend to the provision of a fair and equitable workplace for the team. Increasingly, practices are employing a qualified practice manager who is responsible for the day-to-day enforcement of agreed practice policy to clarify and uphold workplace rights and responsibilities.

Making Clinical Governance work

To take Clinical Governance from concept to reality, personal dental service (PDS) contracts place obligations on the Primary Care Trusts to monitor services though practice visits, and on care providers to provide high quality services.

Defining quality

Quality-focused management techniques place an emphasis on quality in all activities. Now, more than ever, patients are making stringent demands and will not accept poor quality in either the treatment or service aspects of their dental care. As a result, dental businesses need to build quality into their services if they are to succeed. This requires the adoption of a customer focus when designing, planning, implementing, evaluating and auditing services, to ensure they are constantly adapting to patient and team needs whilst observing legislation directives and NHS restructuring.

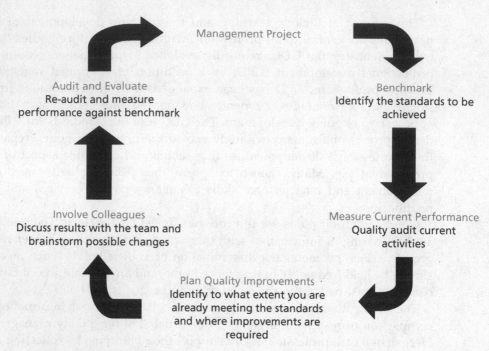

Figure 4.1 Quality cycle.

In addition to being health service providers, general dental practices are small businesses and need to understand the equation between securing income and quality management. To achieve this, managers need to control costs, manage resources and monitor performance. Success in management depends upon the ability to apply the quality cycle, as shown in Figure 4.1.

Principles for total quality management

Total quality management (TQM) first became a key feature of management in the UK during the 1980s. At that time, managers were beginning to recognise the value of basing their company cultures upon quality systems and principles. Over the past 20 years, TQM principles have influenced successful management initiatives, including Clinical Governance.

Clinical Governance is defined as follows:

Total	involving everyone in all company activities
Quality	conforming to requirements
Management	supervision of processes and procedures
TQM	a process for continuous management of quality

. An early version of TQM stems from the work of an American statistician, Dr W Edwards-Deming, who developed a 14-point list defining the Deming philosophy. These 14 points are now regarded as a 'recipe for quality', providing guidance and support for managers and opening the mind to systematic ways of thinking about the purpose of the business, its procedures and processes whilst considering the roles and needs of its people.

Deming's management systems are closely linked to the statistical control of procedures and to establishing clear end results for systems. On a tactical level he advocates that systems be operated on a basis of 'management by positive co-operation', as opposed to management by conflict. In short, this means working in a win–win, rather than a win–lose environment.

The success of TQM is therefore, according to Deming, dependent upon the resolution of conflict and cultivation of teamwork in the workplace. Deming advocates:

'Best efforts are not enough; best efforts will not ensure quality. Everyone putting forth best efforts from their own individual point of view results in much wasted labour; everyone needs to pull in the same direction, the direction which is of the greatest benefit to the company as a whole.'

Another key feature of the Deming philosophy is a concentration on the customer. Many theorists talk about 'satisfying the customer at the lowest possible cost'. Deming, however, writes:

'It will not suffice to have patients that are merely satisfied. An unhappy customer will switch. Unfortunately a satisfied customer may also switch, on the theory that he could not lose much, and may gain. Profit in business comes from repeat patients, patients that boast about your product and service, and that bring their friends with them.'

Clinical Governance, step by step

Under the terms of Clinical Governance, dentists working in the NHS must implement quality assurance measures to ensure:

- All dental care is of consistent quality.
- Effective infection control is maintained.
- Health and safety requirements are satisfied.
- Radiological protection requirements are satisfied.
- The GDC is satisfied in respect of the continuing professional development of dentists.

The principal dentists must appoint a person, usually the practice manager, who is responsible for operating the system. They must display (so that patients can see it) a written practice quality policy and provide an annual report on the quality assurance system to their health authority.

The British Dental Association (BDA) Good Practice Scheme

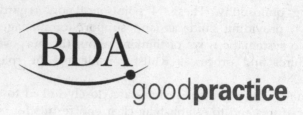

A key role of the BDA is to provide information and guidance to enable its members to excel in the provision of quality dental care. The BDA Good Practice Scheme is widely recognised by the profession as being a baseline for Clinical Governance which will ensure that the services each practice team provides are of high quality. To be included in the Good Practice Scheme, practices are required to meet 96 Standards of which 42 can be demonstrated by the appropriate documents.

Clinical Governance activities
With the overall objectives of Clinical Governance clearly defined as the promotion of quality in dental services, the next step is to clarify what practices need to do for the achievement of these objectives. The required activities fall into three main groups as follows.

Practice management
- Health and safety policies
- Employment policies
- Personal development
- Performer appraisal

Clinical management
- The nine components of Clinical Governance
- Internal governance
- Clinical standards
- Practice and surgery standards
- Team continuing professional development (CPD)

Working with external organisations
- DPB Reference Service, which monitors the quality and probity of NHS treatment claims
- Primary Care Trust (PCT) inspections

Building transparency into quality
Each member of the team should be encouraged to help establish a single practice identity by developing a clear practice vision and by developing

services to achieve it. Every team member should be encouraged to undertake a programme of CPD, to go on courses to learn new skills, and to read dental journals and join professional organisations. In this way staff feel more valued and morale will increase, helping to improve Clinical Governance systems as the team develops. By helping people grow we can ensure effective improvement and the delivery of higher quality services.

Communicating quality to patients

Clinical Governance aims to build public confidence in dental services by ensuring that patients are aware of the measures in place to offer them relevant and effective dental care. Many practices publicise this information by posting their quality charter on their website or including it in their practice information leaflet.

Example Practice Quality Charter
To provide dental care responsive to your needs we will:

(1) Provide dental care of a consistently high quality to all patients and have management systems to define each practice member's responsibilities when looking after you.

(2) In proposing treatment for you we will take your wishes into account and will explain options and costs to enable you to make informed choices between treatment options.

(3) Ask you about your general health and any medication you take, to enable us to treat you safely. All information you provide will be held in confidence.

(4) Ensure your well-being by training every practice member in systems for cross-infection control.

(5) As a matter of routine at your dental assessments we screen for mouth cancer and offer lifestyle advice to minimise the risks of developing this condition.

(6) Review working methods regularly at staff meetings. All staff are encouraged to contribute suggestions for improving our patient care.

(7) Ensure our dentists and registered members of the dental team take part in continuous professional development in line with the General Dental Council's requirements. We aim to keep up to date with current thinking on all aspects of general dentistry, including preventative care, which reduces your need for treatment.

(8) Ensure members of our practice note that dentists are working safely. In the unlikely event that a dentist in this practice becomes unfit to practise, we have systems to guarantee that concerns are investigated and if necessary acted upon.

Clinical Governance is a quality assurance programme for NHS organisations to ensure that patients receive the highest possible quality of care. The aim of Clinical Governance is to put service users' needs first, through effective risk management processes, ensuring dental professionals are qualified and competent to do the work expected of them and by continuously making and documenting improvements to services. Interprofessional teamwork and respect are central to Clinical Governance. The only way we can deliver high quality care and ensure patient safety and comfort is to work collaboratively, valuing one another's contribution.

Chapter 5
Workplace Safety

Dealing with difficult people

A vast range of underlying causes can trigger 'difficult' behaviour from dental patients. In most cases the patients we experience as being 'difficult' are socially well adapted people who have not had their expectations met and are 'having their say' in the hope of getting things put right. By taking an assertive and respectful approach, receptionists can often negotiate a mutually satisfactory outcome. However, there is another group of difficult patients from whom practices must protect their staff. These are people with sociological, psychological or dependency problems, whose behaviour compromises the safety of others.

> During 2004, the British Dental Receptionist Association surveyed its members to find out what kind of patient behaviour left them feeling damaged or abused. They responded that the following three types of behaviour have a detrimental effect on their feelings of well-being.
>
> ■ sarcasm;
> ■ being patronized;
> ■ attribution of blame to staff by patient.

Each of these would be defined as bullying if they took place between colleagues, and employers would have a 'duty of care' to take appropriate remedial action. It is not so straightforward when patients are the bullies.

Under health and safety law, businesses are required to conduct thorough risk assessments and take action to ensure that neither the layout of reception nor agreed working procedures put the well-being of staff or others at risk. When considering how to prevent aggression towards staff, a risk assessment is the initial phase. This should include an analysis of difficult behaviour experienced in the past to define appropriate future prevention measures. Part of this analysis will be the consideration of social, physical and

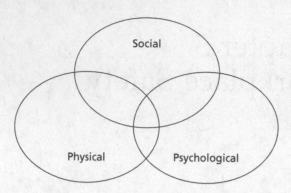

Figure 5.1 The social, physical and psychological influences that combine to affect behaviour.

psychological influences to ascertain how they combine to affect behaviour, as shown in Figure 5.1.

Social influences

Acceptable behaviour differs between social and cultural groups. For example, within some social groups, swearing is accepted as normal everyday language whereas to people from other social groups this type of language can be perceived as aggressive. In the same way, cultural differences lead to misunderstandings as a result of differing cultural norms. Even when the original intentions in cross-culture group communications are amicable, misperceptions shape the response of the receiver and the transaction may take an unintentionally hostile direction.

When the practice defines acceptable language and behaviour and requests compliance, such misunderstandings are reduced. An increasing number of practices give their patients written terms of business in which they explain what patients can expect from the practice and what in exchange the practice expects from its patients. Written in constructive, positive language rather than as a reading of the Riot Act, this creates a businesslike and respectful environment. The terms of business include the practice mission statement and resulting service standards plus a clarification of standards of behaviour expected. An example is as follows.

'At ABC Dental Care we endeavour to deliver the best possible dental services to all of our patients. We will offer help if you need it, provide information when you want it and support if you have concerns about any aspect of your dental well-being. In return we ask you to treat our staff politely. As with all things, occasionally events do not run exactly as we would like them to. We recognise this can be frustrating and could impact on other plans you have made. However, the practice will not tolerate acts of abuse towards its staff and will take action should anyone become verbally or physically abusive to a team member.'

'We want the environment in which you receive your dental care to be safe and welcoming. Your help in achieving this would be very much appreciated.'

We all need to recognise that sometimes people can be rude and inconsiderate, and at times they can be abusive and their behaviour can distress others. This is life. However, if any particular person is a persistent offender, having clarified its position the practice must be prepared to take action to protect the interests of staff.

If people consider they have been unfairly discriminated against, there is every chance they will respond aggressively. In many cases, these responses are the cumulative effect of numerous incidents, and anger is vented as a 'final straw'. Reactions may seem out of proportion, such as that experienced by a receptionist in a practice where a NHS patient pushed over their water dispenser which showed a sign saying, 'This water dispenser is for the use of private patients only'.

When practices take care to ensure that the way they deliver care and services does not discriminate unfairly against any group or groups, the likelihood of such incidents is reduced. However, receptionists may still experience a backlash when conveying the end results of unpopular government health policies to unhappy patients.

Physical influences

When a patient is in physical pain, or is acting on behalf of a partner, child or relative in pain, there is a likelihood of an aggressive response when their needs are not satisfied. People in the UK expect health care to be provided in response to need, and react angrily when refused care.

Drug, substance or alcohol misuse also fuel extreme responses to frustrations. Although such behaviours are obvious risks whilst the person is under the influence, they are less obvious, but equally a threat, when addicts are in withdrawal.

Psychological influences

Fear and anxiety are widely recognised as the cause of stress leading to extreme behaviour. Many people will give highly emotional rather than reasoned responses when under stress. There are a number of reasons why a visit to the dentist is very stressful for many of our patients. Research tells us that their stress is linked to fear of treatment and of being shouted at, and to their perception of lack of control whilst being treated. When looking back over past incidents, it is usually possible to see how a cocktail of these components have fuelled the situation. Even though there are limitations to how we can influence these underlying causes, with an understanding of the cause and effect of each situation in which patients become aggressive we can put measures into place to reduce occurrences and protect staff from feelings of vulnerability and lack of control.

Working with aggressive patients

Dental receptionists say they are becoming increasingly 'stressed-out' from dealing with irate, rude, impatient, emotional, persistent or aggressive people in reception and over the telephone. One key skill required on the front desk is the ability to deal with other people's bad behaviour in an assertive way by offering all reasonable help and support whilst knowing where to draw a line, i.e. when the bad behaviour of others is having a detrimental affect on your well-being.

Growing stress levels, leading to aggressive behaviour, are a problem for society as a whole. In dental practices this phenomenon needs to be approached on three levels:

(1) By agreeing on acceptable standards of patient behaviour, supported by consistent and fair ways for the practice to react to patients who fail to observe them.
(2) By conducting risk assessments to ensure that the practice is doing everything possible to make reception staff safe on the practice premises.
(3) By providing adequate training for reception staff to understand and manage difficult people and situations, enabling them to spot the signs of an escalating situation and to know how to react. In this way confidence is boosted and workplace stress is reduced.

On occasions in which receptionists have experienced frequent problems with difficult patients, a lack of empathy or appropriate training to deal with the emotions has contributed to their problems. They need to recognise the underlying causes when normally polite and reasonable people become 'difficult': because they feel they have been treated unfairly, or their needs have not been satisfied. The four most common patient perceptions of how

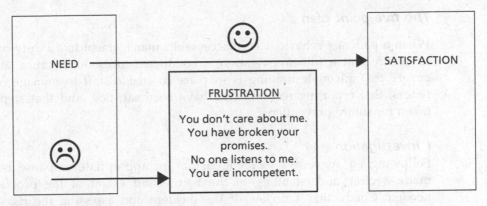

Figure 5.2 Problem recognition and empathy.

the satisfaction of their needs has been frustrated are shown in Figure 5.2. Patients are prepared to do whatever is necessary to make their feelings known: if this means shouting, threatening or taking more extreme measures, then that is what they will do.

Working with angry patients

When patients consider that their needs have been adequately satisfied, they are unlikely to become aggressive. People get angry when they consider that their needs have not been met and believe that you should put this right. At such times it is best to begin by showing recognition of the patient's feelings before problem solving. The receptionist should:

- Use empathy to build trust and show the patient they have made their point. This is achieved by considering how you would feel in their place. If, in this mind-set, you feel their reactions are justified, say, 'I can see why you are not happy. I would feel the same in your position.' In this way you will build rapport and cooperation.
- Listen carefully to what they have to say and give feedback on your understanding of the points they make. In this way you are showing a genuine interest in seeing the situation from their point of view. This respectful approach also allows you to give information and explanations to enable the patient to see things from your point of view, and, if the practice is in any way at fault, to identify remedial action.
- Be solution- rather than problem-focused. Be positive. If you cannot do exactly what the patient wants, outline what you can do and offer alternatives. Never emphasise what you cannot do; rather stress what you could do. For example, don't say, 'I cannot give you a filling appointment after 5 pm.' Do say, 'I can give you our latest filling appointment at 5.30, or an early morning appointment at 8 am.'

Most people will respond positively when treated with respect and consideration.

The five-point plan

When a patient's behaviour is unacceptable, management has a duty of care to ensure that a full investigation is conducted to establish cause, and to ensure that adequate training is in place to enable staff to manage occurrences, that reporting requirements have been satisfied, and that steps are taken for future prevention.

I Investigation

Following an aggressive incident, before an appropriate response can be made a clear understanding of the nature and extent of the problem is needed. Conducting a review of the incident and assessing the risks will achieve this. The aim of the review is to highlight areas of need and facilitate the design of strategies for future prevention.

Investigation for effective problem solving requires identification of root causes rather than effects. The simplest way to delve into the root causes of problems is to ask the 'Five Whys'. For example:

(1) Why did the person become difficult?
     Because she was angry and completely lost it.
(2) Why was she angry?
     She was kept waiting and then couldn't get what she wanted.
(3) Why was she kept waiting?
     We were short-staffed.
(4) Why were we short-staffed?
     Because the management never plans for school half-term.
(5) Why didn't we have what she wanted?
     We didn't anticipate the demand or check our supply.

Common sense? In this real example the practice's initial reaction was to find ways to increase security following an assault – in other words to deal with the symptoms rather than the causes of the problem. After considering the 'Five Whys' they were able to recognise which preventative actions they needed to take.

II Training

At times you may well have problems dealing with your own stress levels. If at such times you find yourself in a tricky situation, your untrained and unprepared reactions may be inappropriate. For risks that cannot be controlled, procedures must be in place and staff trained to follow them.

Training aims

- To make staff aware of potential risks and preventative measures.
- To enable staff to identify threatening situations at their earliest stages.
- To clarify safe reactions to threatening situations.
- To familiarise staff with practice policy and procedures.

Training objectives

The team will be able to take appropriate and reasoned steps to ensure their own safety and the safety of others from aggression in the workplace. Practices have a legal duty to implement safe work systems which do not put staff at risk, and to provide training for the following:

(a) *Handling aggressive incidents*. Staff should be trained in the following skills when dealing with an aggressor:

- Use of assertive non-verbal language. Body language makes up a staggering 80% of all communication. Without saying a word you can set the tone of an interaction through body language. An assertive 'I'm OK, you're OK' approach is communicated with relaxed gestures, eye contact and tone of voice. By remaining assertive you can influence the path of events. The aggression will escalate out of control when both parties use aggressive non-verbal language
- Encourage the potential aggressor to talk. In most cases the aggressor wants to make their feelings known. The more difficult this is made for them, the more force they will use. By giving them the opportunity to talk and be heard, you reduce the need for them to use force to make their point.
- Give reassurance that you are working for a win–win outcome. Having listened to the aggressor's point of view, you should give clear messages that you are ready to do whatever, within the bounds of possibility, will bring about a satisfactory outcome. In this way you are making a clear statement that whatever the patient's problem is, you are part of the solution, rather than part of the problem.
- Proceed gradually. Although your instincts tell you to get away from this threatening situation, you should not give the aggressor the impression that you are rushing them. Make them feel you will give the matter the time it requires to reach a mutually agreeable solution.
- Anticipate violence. Do not leave yourself open or vulnerable to attack. Try to maintain at least an arm's length between you and the aggressor, giving you the chance to sidetrack any blow the aggressor may deliver.
- Avoid audiences, but do not isolate yourself with the aggressor. Some aggressors thoroughly enjoy being the focus of attention and will play to an audience in the staffroom. Although you do not want to give them the chance to play to the crowd, it is never advisable to isolate yourself with anyone displaying signs of or threatening aggression. If a situation is likely to get out of hand, move out of the reception area but make sure you are not putting yourself at risk by being alone with someone aggressive. The practice should have a policy for relocating potentially aggressive incidents, developed in line with health and safety requirements.

(b) *Talking with the aggressor*. Good communication skills form the basis for mutually satisfactory outcomes. When handling aggressive incidents, communication begins with reactive listening skills and progresses on to proactive problem-solving skills. Training should enable staff to:

- Break the issues down into component parts. This is part of the investigation process in which the patient gives a full and frank outline of the problem from their point of view so that each aspect can be identified. This is part of the 'talking it through' process designed to build trust and confidence.
- Offer alternatives. Being given alternatives reduces feelings of loss of control over situations. Even if none of the alternatives is ideal, the aggressor will be able to see that you are doing all you can to find a solution that meets their needs.
- Give them time to make their decisions. Rather than asking for a decision on the spot, allow them time to consider their options and get back to you with their answer. Don't leave the timespan open-ended; give them a time by which you must have a decision.
- Present both sides of the argument. Show the aggressor that there are valid reasons why you cannot fully meet their expectations. When people can understand why, they are more likely to be compliant.

III Post-incident support

Following aggressive incidents, employers have a duty to provide the staff involved with:

- *Understanding* – to recognise what has happened and why, and to adjust to it.
- *Comfort* – to talk about the incident and overcome the feelings of loss of control and self-blame enabling staff to regain confidence and return to normal working patterns.
- *Warmth* – in some cases the member of staff may be in shock and need to restore their body temperature. At the very least they will need time to relax and explore the way forward.

Some people are better than others when it comes to dealing with difficult people; they seem to have been born with natural energy and confidence whereas others must work for it.

IV Reporting

An accurate account of events should be completed as soon as possible after the event and agreed with all persons present. Under RIDDOR 95 (The Reporting of Injuries, Diseases and Dangerous Occurrences Regulations 1995), employers are required to report cases in which employees have been off work for three days or more following an assault that has resulted in physical injury.

In addition to being a legal requirement, reporting is essential in a world in which we are increasingly held accountable for both our action and our inaction. It is also difficult to manage violence effectively and focus resources unless information is shared and recorded.

Two of the most common problems faced by managers tackling violence are:

■ under-reporting of incidents;
■ poor quality reporting.

Many staff view reporting an incident as pointless, feeling that it is unlikely to be followed up or that little will change as a result. Some do not understand the process or are afraid of drawing attention to themselves; others simply find it difficult to find the time to write a report during the shift and don't want to wait behind after work. There is also a belief in some practices that it is best to say as little as possible concerning the actual events that took place. When staff experience abuse on a regular basis, they can come to accept the situation and stop reporting. Where a member of staff feels it is impractical to report every incident of verbal abuse, they should at least be encouraged to report incidents that they or others present may have found threatening.

V Future prevention

Where assaults or threats occur, post-incident procedures may well make the difference between a person returning to work quickly having come to terms with events, or finding it difficult or impossible to return to work. A management process needs to be put in place to ensure supportive post-incident responses. Although there may be time difficulties surrounding debriefing processes, this should not be an excuse for inaction. Initiatives can arise from the debrief process to instigate proactive measures for the prevention of potentially traumatic events including:

■ Education as to:
  – the effects of violent or other traumatic events;
  – personal coping strategies and peer support;
  – post-incident procedures and sources of support.
■ The creation of:
  – the procedure immediately following an incident;
  – follow-up and long-term support strategies;
  – confidence restoration programmes;
  – legal advice and support;
  – learning mechanisms and feedback loop.

Criminal acts towards dental receptionists are often spurred by patients' discontentment about life in general, directed at a 'soft target': someone who will not retaliate. Verbal abuse such as shouting, swearing and sarcasm are everyday experiences for many receptionists. As a result, practices have growing problems recruiting receptionists. Although prevention is the ideal way of managing aggression, practices must provide guidance for dealing with threatening situations in a policy for managing aggression.

Health and safety

The first health and safety legislation in this country came into force in 1802 to protect workers in the textile industry. Between 1802 and 1974 the range and scope of health and safety legislation gradually increased, until massive changes were made with the introduction of the Health and Safety at Work Act (HASWA) 1974.

The need for a new consultative approach to occupational health and safety was recognised following several major disasters, including the Aberfan disaster of 1966. The HASWA 1974 was introduced to provide a broad framework within which health and safety could be regulated by providing comprehensive systems for dealing with the health, safety and welfare of people at work and of members of the public affected by their work activities.

In 1972 Lord Robens was appointed to review all existing health and safety regulations. The Robens Committee reached a number of interesting conclusions. They found the existing laws were confusing and contradictory, with overlapping jurisdiction between enforcement bodies. As a result there was apathy towards day-to-day implementation of safety rules. The HASWA set out legal obligations and placed a duty of care on both employers and employees, to be enforced though a unified administration.

Running a business safely and without risks to health makes sense; in the end it saves time, money and a lot of heartache. In their report the Robens Committee noted that existing legislation did little to encourage employers to improve conditions beyond the minimum standards. The Committee believed a self-regulation approach would encourage employers to recognise the value of good standards of health and safety within their businesses.

The Robens Committee emphasised the importance of clear communication between employers and employees about health and safety. To this end they recommended that formal statements of safety policy should be a requirement and that a systematic hazard assessment should be carried out. They placed the following duties upon employers, employees, the self-employed, manufacturers and suppliers.

Employers
- To safeguard, as far as reasonably practicable, the health, safety and welfare of the workforce. (This re-states employers' duty of care under civil law, in particular requiring the provision of safe equipment and systems of work.)
- To provide a statement of safety policy and bring it to the attention of the workforce.
- To inform employees about safety matters on a right-to-know basis.
- To train employees in safe working practices.

Employers have similar duties to others, including contractors and the general public.

Employees
- To take reasonable care of themselves and others.
- To co-operate with the employer in safety matters.

Manufacturers/suppliers
- To ensure that any substance or article provided is safe when used properly, and to provide instructions to allow safe usage.

As a result of the findings of the Robens Committee the HASWA 1974 established new methods of occupational health and safety and 'enabled' new ways of introducing future safety legislation. The Act:

- completely renovated and modernised existing health and safety law;
- placed new general duties on all persons involved in work activities;
- provided new powers and penalties for the enforcement of safety laws.

Enforcement

The Health and Safety Executive (HSE) was set up to enforce this legislation. Their inspectors are empowered to access and inspect any workplace and can take the following actions if the HASWA is being contravened:

- seize and remove unsafe equipment;
- issue a dated Improvement Notice;
- issue a Prohibition Notice;
- prosecute under the HASWA or criminal law;
- issue verbal and/or written instructions, which are less formal.

European health and safety directives

The biggest shake-up in health and safety legislation since 1974 was the introduction of the six-pack. This legislation was introduced in all European States in 1992, coming into effect on 1 January 1993. The six-pack consisted of six health and safety regulations the aim of which was to set the parameters for the management of workplace health and safety.

What is the six-pack?

The six-pack was issued by the European Commission and introduced in Britain through six European Directives. Its main regulation is the Management of Health and Safety at Work Regulations 1999, also known as the 'Management Regs'. These first came into force in 1993 and were updated in 1999. Another placed a legal duty on employers to carry out risk assessments as a first step towards ensuring a safe workplace. Other 'six-pack' regulations cover heating, lighting and ventilation at work; the safe use of computer screens and keyboards; handling heavy or awkward loads; rest breaks; and personal protective equipment.

Dental practice health and safety

New working procedures for health and safety in dental practice are introduced on a regular basis and are supported with policy updates from reliable sources such as the BDA and the Confederation of Dental Employers (CODE). This book will review general regulations that aim to create a preventative approach to workplace safety by ensuring workplaces are:

- clean;
- safe;
- ergonomically aware;
- risk assessed;
- risk managed;
- hazard free.

Prevention

Each of the above has a shared aim. An important function of health and safety is accident prevention. What do you understand by the term 'accident'? Here are some suggestions:

- an unplanned event resulting in injury, for example cuts, bruises, fractures, burns;
- something that happens as a result of human error;
- an unforeseeable event that could not have been prevented;
- an undesired happening resulting in emotional or physical harm;
- an uncontrolled situation that results in harm to a person.

Leading on from the above here are some other points to consider, thereby broadening the definition of accidents and the concept of health and safety:

- an unplanned event resulting in ill health, for example: back problems, eye strain, hearing loss, occupational asthma, blood poisoning;

- an uncontrolled situation resulting in property/equipment damage;
- an undesired happening that causes business interruption;
- an unexpected event that could have been prevented.

There are fundamental differences between the first group of suggestions. Spillage of a chemical could result in burns to the skin: the effects are recognised immediately. However, if we broaden the definition we see that inhalation of the same chemical may result in occupational asthma in which the effects are delayed for many years; both could result from the same accident. The first suggestions also focus on someone to blame – there is reference to 'human error' – and there are misconceptions that the event could not have been prevented.

With prevention at the heart of health and safety regulations, practices must produce a health and safety policy to clarify and communicate safety measures to everyone affected by the work of the business.

Health and safety policy

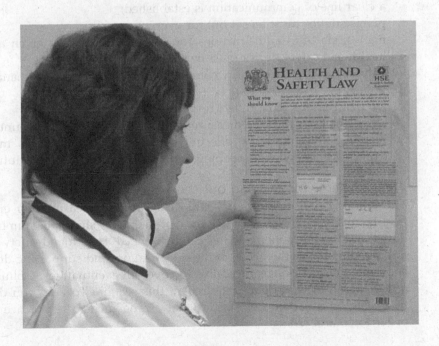

The practice's health and safety policy must be user friendly and a 'live', working *aide-mémoire*. It must be part of the practice policy and comprise: a statement of commitment; organisation and designation of responsibilities; and arrangements for carrying out the policy.

A statement of commitment
This should include commitments to:

- safeguard the health and safety of all persons;
- comply with health and safety legislation relevant to the work activities;
- information, instruction and training for the team;
- managers' responsibility for supervising work;
- arrangements for consultation with the team;
- provide for competent people to assist the employer;
- monitor, review and revise where appropriate.

The most senior partner should sign and date the statement. An issue number is useful when revising the policy. It should also outline employees' general commitments.

Organisation
This describes how responsibilities are designated:

- structure and responsibilities are laid down for implementing health and safety at all levels;
- a clear line of communication is established;
- precise duties must be set out for everyone;
- names, job titles and functions for employees who are given additional health and safety duties must be stated;
- employers must appoint a competent person to assist in managing the policy;
- job descriptions must reflect responsibilities;
- responsibilities must be measured and evaluated (this is accountability);
- responsibilities must be effectively designated (individuals must have experience, knowledge, training and skills to carry out their duties).

Arrangements for carrying out the policy
The working part of the policy will detail specific measures for ensuring a healthy and safe workplace. Each page of the policy should be numbered and dated; in this way policy updates can be tracked. Health and safety activities must be tailored to the needs of the organisation, and supporting documents should set out working procedures to cover all eventualities. Opinion varies about the amount of detail required in this section. To help you determine how lengthy it should be, decide what arrangements the practice needs in order to control risks.

Policy circulation and distribution
Developing the policy is the first step in the communication between employer and employee. Team attitudes towards their own and other people's health and safety impact on safety standards, as do attitudes of management. Therefore, effective communication between both is essential if the policy is to work for you.

How do you communicate the practice policy?
Here are some suggestions:

- Issue a copy to new recruits prior to commencing employment.
- Include a copy with contracts of employment.
- Include related duties in job descriptions.
- Review each section of the policy with staff as part of their induction.
- Discuss the arrangements and events at each practice meeting.
- Post regular reminders and memory joggers.
- Display posters and notices.
- Insert updates with pay slips.
- Discuss compliance as part of annual staff appraisal.
- Health and safety are everyone's concern and depend upon cooperation and commitment of both employers and employees.

Occupational health

The 2001 UK census revealed that 10% of the population believed their health was 'not good'. A quarter of the UK population were smokers, one-fifth were obese and one-fifth reported suffering from stress at work. Furthermore, deaths related to alcohol consumption more than doubled between 1980 and 2000 in England and Wales. It is little wonder that most practice managers consider that managing staff absence is one of their biggest challenges. This being the case the concept of wellness management, which is producing excellent results in larger corporations throughout the world, could prove to be a worthwhile initiative when scaled down to relevant dental businesses.

Wellness management is about helping people to look and feel better and to be physically well. The approach focuses on prevention rather than cure in the belief that a healthier workforce is happier and more productive in the long term. The approach brings together well people and consistent good management to create a 'well company'. Instead of managing the effects of staff sick leave, companies can prevent employees from becoming sick.

Practices have to compete for staff within a labour market in which attracting the right calibre of staff may be close to impossible. When employers can offer tangible fringe benefits, they become a more attractive prospect to potential employees. Meaningful health management initiatives can be seen as both a good business investment and a way to compete with other employers for the cream of the crop in the job market. Coupled with the fact that people who are stressed or constantly ill through their jobs are more likely to leave, wellness management becomes an attractive prospect.

Another reason to follow a wellness plan is the employer's duty of care since UK and EU legislation obliges employers to look at the physical as well as the psychological well-being of staff. Duty of care aside, some employers simply care about their workforce and have wellness programmes in place that consider the whole team.

Designing a wellness initiative

In primary dental care, the concept of preventing dental disease is central to our culture. This concept can be extended to the general health of the staff in respect of preventable conditions, with lifestyle links such as diet, smoking and stress. Such programmes will meet with resistance if presented in a way perceived as intrusive upon individuals' rights to choose their lifestyle. Programmes should be presented as opportunities to access health management resources. For example, Standard Life Healthcare has given employees access to a personalised, private, on-line service where their health and lifestyles can be analysed and where advice on nutrition, sleep, stress and exercise is available. They have introduced 'free fruit days' and give staff nutritional bars every month. Seminars promoting healthy eating and relaxation are held and the company has introduced subsidised on-site massages. These initiatives were well accepted and exercise classes were requested. The results were impressive, with a 22.5% decrease in staff turnover in the first year of the programme and a 4.9% cut in absences. Standard Life is convinced that, because people are feeling better about their health, productivity is improving.

Developing a scheme relevant to your practice will take management and investment. One approach would be to offer health care insurance as part of the employment package. Companies such as Norwich Union offer private medical insurance, an online personalised health management service and a 24-hour GP helpline and stress counselling.

Now that we have adopted continuous professional development in our professional lives, we are now ready to add personal development initiatives by including health. Discussing well-being topics in practice staff meetings will enable the team to investigate a range of health and relaxation programmes.

Alongside work to promote the health of staff, creating a fair and equitable management culture in which people and companies can thrive is the second component to wellness. Chronic tiredness is a massive problem in workplaces where staff shortages and excessive demand for services exist side by side. Practices must be realistic in their expectations of staff and use management processes to protect them from having unrealistic expectations placed upon them.

With as many as 50% of public sector and FTSE-500 companies saying they will have wellness managers in post by the end of 2007, they must be convinced of the potential benefits. People have the same health needs; we need to find ways of meeting those needs irrespective of the size of our organisations.

Worrying about stress?

Working in the dental profession is widely acknowledged as being a relatively stressful way to earn a living. All members of the dental team are subjected to stressful workplace situations. The Health and Safety Executive (HSE) has always worked to promote acceptable standards of physical and environmental safety in the workplace. The improvement notice, in respect of employee stress levels, that has been served on West Dorset Hospitals NHS Trust is proof that stress is a safety issue. Measures to combat psychosocial stressors will be included in the HSE's action plan for achieving its target of reducing by one-third the number of days lost through ill health by 2011.

Some sources of work-related stress cannot be completely eliminated, such as stressors related to the nature of the work, demands to make changes for safety reasons, or the need to enable the business to compete and survive. In such cases it is important to manage the change process. This involves creating adequate and respectful communication channels to clearly explain the rationale for changes and to demonstrate that the aims are, in the long run, to ensure a happy, healthy and productive dental team.

There are standards in place to enable employers to plan measures to prevent employee stress from costing the business in terms of employee downtime or action taken against the employer by the HSE. The standards cover:

- demands;
- control;
- support;
- relationships;
- roles;
- change.

In each of these areas communication is the key. A review of practice policy is advisable as well as monitoring processes to ensure that your practice policies are consistently enforced. You need to perform reviews with the following information in mind related to each draft standard.

Demands

The practice has achieved the draft standard if at least 85% of the team say they are able to cope with the demands of their job and that systems are in place to respond to any concerns they may have.

This means that employers must ensure that work demands placed on employees are achievable. Particular attention needs to be paid to covering long-term sickness or maternity leave if employees are expected to cover for absent colleagues over long periods of time. Another consideration is whether workers and their supervisors have the necessary skills and competences for work tasks. To ensure appropriate skills are in place, employers are wise to invest in team training leading to recognised qualifications.

The 'demands standard' also highlights the physical working environment and the need to undertake risk assessments and provide ways for staff to raise their concerns about health and safety issues.

Control

The practice has achieved the draft standard if 85% of the team are consulted about the way they work and that systems are in place to respond to their concerns.

To meet this standard, team members should be encouraged and supported in developing new skills through training and development measures and using their new skills in their work. Such measures could be in-house development initiatives such as inductions and appraisals or team training sessions as well as recognised formal qualifications.

Support

The practice has achieved the draft standard if 85% of the team say that colleagues and superiors support them and that systems are in place to respond to their concerns.

To meet this standard, we need to create an environment in which it feels safe to admit to having a problem with particular aspects of your work. The practice should then provide training and support to strengthen areas of weakness. It is also an opportunity to evaluate the related systems and procedures.

Relationships

The practice has achieved the draft standard if 55% of the team say that they do not experience unacceptable behaviour (e.g. bullying) at work and that systems are in place to respond to their concerns.

There may be individuals in the team who fail to see eye to eye for whatever reason. It is vital that the practice sets out its expectations for team interactions and enforces them equitably.

Twenty per cent of workers interviewed in research commissioned by the HSE said they were stressed by workplace relationships. Small dental teams are more at risk from this type of work stress and the practice must be very clear about its role and objectives in dealing with interpersonal problems between employees or between managers and workers.

Roles

The practice has achieved the draft standard if 55% of the team say that they understand their role and responsibilities and that systems are in place to respond to their concerns.

To meet this standard it is vital that work roles are communicated and consistent. Not only should individuals be clear about their own role and status in the practice; team members should also have a clear understanding of their colleagues' roles and responsibilities.

Change

The practice has achieved the draft standard if 55% of the team say that they are consulted about organisational changes and that systems are in place to respond to their concerns.

To meet this standard requires regular staff meetings, no matter how informal, provided they are recognised as being a part of the team communication/consultation process and are recorded as having taken place. In particular, the content should cover how any changes will impact on individuals and give some form of timetable for the changes.

During the 18th and 19th centuries there were frequent deaths and injuries in the unregulated workplace. Although daunting, health and safety legislation clearly has a massive impact, preventing people from being harmed as a result of workplace activities.

Cross-infection control

Cross-infection is the transmission of disease from one person to another, both in the treatment rooms and on the front desk from the patient to any member of the dental team, or vice versa. To ensure that cross-infection is prevented, every member of the team must be aware of potential cross-infection risks and know how to avoid them. The practice must follow a policy of Universal Infection Control, so described because its measures aim to protect *all* people affected by the practice's activities.

Universal Infection Control routines involve a range of procedures, as follows.

Sterilisation

Sterilisation involves the use of heat, chemicals or radiation to destroy all germs. Any instruments contaminated with oral and other body fluids must be sterilised after use. The first phase of this process is pre-sterilisation cleaning, such as scrubbing, using chemical disinfectants or an ultrasonic bath. The second phase of sterilisation is autoclaving. Autoclaves work by killing microbes with superheated steam and are used for instruments such as: tweezers, mouth mirrors and numerous other hand instruments; burs (the small drill bits that do the actual cutting of the tooth); metal cups; trays on which the instruments are placed; dental handpieces (drills).

The only instruments not autoclaved are those used once and then thrown away. These include: needles, scalpel blades, saliva ejectors (suction tips), napkins, towels and cups.

Barriers

Clinical staff routinely wear gloves, masks, goggles or face shields during treatment. These serve as protective barriers against the transmission of germs. The need to operate barriers against the transmission of germs extends to the front desk, where staff should be trained to recognise potential risks and take preventative measures such as the following.

- *Vaccinations.* All staff, including administrators, should be vaccinated against rubella, poliomyelitis, pertussis, diphtheria, tuberculosis, tetanus and hepatitis B.
- *Handling infected materials.* Never accept used tissues from patients. These should be treated as contaminated waste and disposed of in a yellow waste bag and not as uncontaminated office or kitchen waste.
- *Receiving dentures from patients.* Always wear gloves to handle patients' dentures.

Chemical disinfectants

After every treatment the nurse ensures that the dental chair and working surfaces are wiped with disinfectant chemicals. Impressions and work to be forwarded to labs are also disinfected and packed carefully, to protect the work and reduce the risk of cross-infection from surgery to reception and the lab. Between patients, clinical staff wash their hands with antiseptic soap. Reception staff are well advised to wash their hands with antiseptic soap at the end of each shift on reception.

Disposal of waste

Practices are required to segregate clinical and non-clinical waste. Clinical waste is waste contaminated with blood, saliva or other body fluids, which must be placed in a clinical waste sack and stored with due regard for health and safety on practice premises until collected by a licensed carrier for disposal by high temperature incineration. Clinical waste sacks must never be more than three-quarters full, the air must be squeezed out to avoid bursting when handled, and they must be tied at the neck. Used sharps (needles and surgical blades) must be sealed in UN-approved puncture-proof containers. Sharps containers should be disposed of when two-thirds full. When waste is collected for incineration, a transfer note must be signed by both parties and kept for two years.

The term 'special waste' is used for the disposal of prescribed medicines, irritants, and harmful, toxic, carcinogenic or corrosive waste. Disposal of special waste is subject to more stringent controls than clinical waste; records and receipts must be kept for three years.

Uncontaminated office paper waste should be stored separately from general kitchen and household waste and disposed of at a local recycling centre. See Figure 5.3.

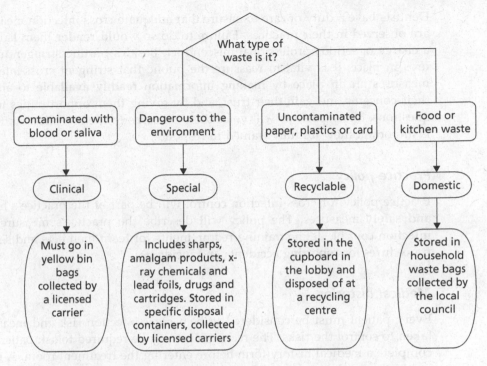

Figure 5.3 Practice waste disposal.

Cross-infection measures on reception

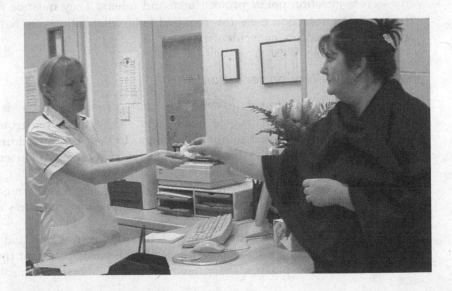

Dentists have a duty of care to ensure that adequate cross-infection measures are observed in their practices. Failure to do so would render them liable to a charge of serious professional misconduct. Besides putting stringent measures in place, it is vital to reassure the public that stringent cross-infection measures are in place by making information readily available to answer their concerns and gain their trust, and by giving them opportunities to ask questions. Many patients will voice their concerns to the reception staff so it is important they are fully trained to respond.

Practice policy

Practice policy for cross-infection control will be part of the practice's health and safety measures. The policy will describe the practice's measures for infection control, define training requirements for team members and set out procedures for reporting accidents and incidents.

Medical histories

Every patient must be considered to be a cross-infection risk and measures taken to control the risks. The receptionist may be required to ask patients to complete a medical history form before entering the treatment room. A medical history update is required at every appointment to ensure every possible measure is taken for the protection of patients and the dental team.

Training

All dental staff should be aware of their role in infection control. Training should equip the team to understand how the measures outlined in the practice's cross-infection policy protect them and others. They must be aware of the personal protection measures required, and what actions are required in the event of accidents or incidents.

Wearing jewellery on reception

Studies have demonstrated that the skin underneath rings is a risk factor as it harbours bacteria. Practice health and safety measures require that dental team members wear minimal jewellery. In the case of wedding rings, careful hand washing measures should be taken to remove bacteria from under rings.

Regular accidents and incident reviews, including near misses, must be discussed in team meetings to ensure that the 'best practice' measures are kept up to date.

Infection control in dentistry is subject to ongoing research and debate. Implementing realistic safety measures needs the participation of the whole dental team. Every practice must have an agreed infection control policy, developed with consideration of each team member's needs and subjected to regular reviews.

The dental profession has always taken precautions to prevent cross-infection. Indeed, with new knowledge and better technology, the procedures to prevent infection have become extremely effective. Where a programme of Universal Infection Control is observed, incidents of cross-infection are practically nil.

Chapter 6
Using the Appointment Book

Booking treatments

The appointment book is central to reception services and an essential tool for practice management. A well planned and managed appointment system streamlines services, and is characterised by timely treatments with few delays for patients or clinicians. The aims of the appointment system are to enable every member of the team to plan and prepare for their work, and to ensure that clinicians and patients are available at the appointed time with the necessary equipment to hand. An undisciplined appointment system creates chaos.

The appointment book defines the workload for each day and must be governed by agreed rules for booking treatments. Receptionists must be aware of the needs of the treatment rooms, labs and patients, to ensure that these are taken into account when appointments are booked. They need to know if each appointment is a 'stand-alone' appointment, to be booked whenever the required amount of time is available, or if there is a need to coordinate appointments with more than one clinician. In some cases considerations in respect of lab turnaround times or the availability of specialist equipment will influence the appointments given.

An effective appointments system requires cooperation between patients and the dental team. When patients fail to keep their appointments, valuable time is lost for which most practices will require reimbursement before another appointment is booked. The smooth running of the appointment system is also compromised when patients arrive to find the receptionist has failed to enter their appointment accurately in the appointment book. At best this results in delays for subsequent patients, when their dentist 'fits them in'; at worst, the frustration of a wasted journey provokes an angry response from patients.

For dental businesses time is money, so when appointments are missed there is a cost involved. Reception procedures can make a considerable impact on whether patients attend for their appointments. Research shows that the new patient's assessment and initial treatment appointments are the ones most likely be missed. Practice managers should therefore develop patient-focused reception services to welcome new patients to the practice and ensure that their first experiences lay down the foundations of a respectful and enduring relationship. Reception staff must be well trained in new patient procedures, which should be reinforced with clear working instructions to ensure consistency and reduce mistakes.

What you need to know when booking appointments

When receptionists are aware of surgery procedures, they are better able to book appropriate appointments. Practices have a duty to be clear about all aspects of the treatments prescribed for patients. To avoid misunderstandings, terms of business should be clarified when new patients first contact the practice, and reinforced as necessary when appointments are booked. The receptionist should:

- clarify whether services are offered on an NHS or private basis;
- explain what will happen during the appointment;
- specify all costs and payment requirements.

Clinicians are responsible for ensuring that patients are well informed about and give informed consent to treatment. It is nevertheless important that the receptionist reinforces certain messages when booking appointments, for example by reminding patients to eat before attending for long treatment appointments.

Some long treatments require intensive concentration from clinicians so should not be booked in close succession. Most dentists prefer to have quick, routine appointments booked directly after long or intricate treatment appointments.

Working instructions

In every practice clear working instructions for operating the appointment system should be readily available to equip any member of the team to cover for reception duties if necessary. This chapter will outline generalised information and provide alphabetical guidance for booking appointments, and on treatment room considerations.

Considerations when booking appointments

Air abrasion
This is a technique for removing diseased tooth tissue or staining, by driving finely graded aluminium oxide powder and compressed air through a very fine tip. It can be used as an alternative to the high-speed drill, and, as there is no need for anaesthesia, procedures can often be completed in less time (Table 6.1).

Table 6.1 Air abrasion: considerations.

Needs to be considered	
Treatment room	If this technique is not frequently used in your practice, try to book air abrasion appointments at the end of the session, to allow preparation time. These appointments should not be booked in rapid succession to each other, to allow time for cross-infection control of limited equipment resources.
Patient	The patient should be given a clear idea of how long they will spend in the treatment room and what to expect after the appointment. A written treatment plan, an estimate of cost and payment requirements should be provided when booking appointments.

Assessment/recall

In the past this procedure was referred to as an examination or check-up. Today assessment is the preferred terminology, as it represents the true nature of this procedure during which past, current and future treatment needs of the teeth and oral soft tissues are ascertained. Unless the patient is an expectant mother or there are other reasons why x-rays cannot be taken, the initial assessment will include intra- and extraoral x-rays.

Dental x-rays provide a picture of teeth and mouth. X-rays are passed through the tissues of the mouth and on to a film where it forms an image. Structures that are dense (such as silver fillings or metal restoration) will block most of the x-rays and appear as a clear patch on developed film. Structures containing air will be black on film, and teeth, tissue and fluid will appear as shades of grey.

An x-ray enables the dentist to check the health status in places that cannot otherwise be seen such as in between teeth, and below the gum margins. An x-ray will also show unerupted teeth so that the dentist can plan to prevent future problems, such as those linked to impacted wisdom teeth.

New patients

The receptionist needs to be aware of numerous treatment and business considerations for booking a new patient. When booking a new patient assessment, a receptionist could say the following to the patient:

> 'On your first visit we will carry out a full assessment of your mouth. This will establish what treatment you've had in the past and your present treatment needs. Unless there is any reason not to, we will take a full set of radiographs to complete your oral assessment. This will take around 30 minutes and the cost will be £45.00, payable by card on booking your appointment.'

Table 6.2 Assessment/recall: considerations.

Needs to be considered	
Treatment room	Many practices book 30 minutes for an initial assessment. For existing patients assessment appointments may be shorter as per established practice procedures. When booking, ask the patient if they have any dental problems or concerns and make this information available to the dentist at the time of the assessment. Many dentists prefer to see assessment patients between their treatment appointments.
Patient	Ask if the patient has any concerns or special needs for which provision will need to be made. Post a welcome pack out to new patients, outlining practice services, showing how to find the practice, explaining cancellation protocols and confirming the appointment.

It is advisable to send patients a welcome pack by post, in which they are given details of the practice and your standard terms of business.

Existing patients
Dentists will make recommendations to individual patients about how often they should attend for regular assessments. Some practices send recalls to patients, whereas others rely on patients remembering to book their routine appointments. In most cases recalls are sent out on a monthly basis (Table 6.2).

Bridges
Dental bridges are used to fill gaps made by missing teeth. Every dental bridge will be designed by the dentist to meet the patient's particular dental needs. There are a number of designs for dental bridges, all of which involve fusing a prosthetic tooth, usually between two porcelain crowns. In most cases there will be two crowns at either end of the bridge, cemented on to the teeth either side of the missing tooth. Bridges are cemented into place and unlike partial dentures cannot be removed by the patient.

For traditional bridges two appointments are needed, the first to prepare the tooth and take impressions, which are sent to the laboratory where the bridge will be made by a dental technician, and the second a week or two later for the bridge to be fitted. Once the teeth have been prepared, a temporary crown will be placed over the teeth to protect them until the bridge has been received from the laboratory (Table 6.3).

Crowns
A crown can make a tooth stronger, improve its appearance, or cover and support a tooth with a large filling when very little natural tooth is left.

Table 6.3 Bridges: considerations.

Needs to be considered	
Treatment room	To ensure the finished work is of the highest possible standard, it is advisable to forward impressions to the dental lab on the day they are taken. Book appointments at such times to ensure the impressions will be ready to catch that day's post or lab collection schedule. Although much of the equipment required will be fairly standard, special diamond burs may be required. When booking the patient's 'fit' appointment, to make sure the lab work is back in time most practices request the lab to return work at least one day before.
Patient	The patient should be given a clear idea of how long they will spend in the treatment room on each visit. The patient should be informed that temporary crowns will be fitted while the lab is constructing their bridge. Details of payment requirements should be clarified when booking the appointments. Payment should be collected to ensure the laboratory invoices are always covered before the work is fitted.

Crowns can protect weak teeth from breaking, or restore one that is already broken. They can be used to cover teeth that are discoloured or misshapen, or to cover dental implants.

For traditional crowns, two appointments are needed, the first to prepare the tooth and take impressions, which are sent to the laboratory where the crown will be made by a dental technician. The second appointment should be a week or two later for the crown to be fitted. Once the tooth has been prepared, a temporary crown will be placed over the tooth to protect it until the new crown has been received from the laboratory.

There are a number of types of crown available. The materials of choice will depend on clinical and cost considerations. The most popular choices of materials for crowns are:

- porcelain;
- porcelain bonded to gold or precious metal;
- gold.

In some practices, new high-tech systems are available such as CEREC, where crowns are manufactured at the practice whilst the patient is in the dental chair. In this case only one appointment is required (Table 6.4).

Dentures
The dentist or clinical dental technician designs every denture to meet the individual needs of the patient. Dentures are used to replace lost or missing

Table 6.4 Crowns: considerations.

Needs to be considered	
Treatment room	When booking the appointment, consideration should be given to forwarding the impressions to the lab quickly to prevent distortion due to deterioration of the impression materials as they dry out. Crown preps should not be booked in rapid succession to each other. If the crown is being manufactured at the practice, one visit only is required. Otherwise the 'crown fit' appointment should be made at a time which will ensure that the finished crown will be available in the practice.
Patient	The patient should be given a clear idea of how long they will spend in the treatment room on each visit. They need to be aware that their mouth will be numb for a short while after the appointment and that a temporary crown will be in place after the first appointment until the 'fit' appointment. Details of payment requirements should be clarified when booking the appointments. From the financial point of view, the crown should be fitted as soon as possible after it is returned from the lab to ensure that the patient has paid for it before the lab invoices the practice.

teeth to enable patients with missing teeth to eat, speak and smile with confidence. A full denture is one which replaces all of the natural teeth in either the upper or lower jaws. This is shown on the patient's records as F/– for a full upper denture, –/F for a full lower and F/F for upper and lower. A partial denture fills in the spaces created by lost or missing teeth and is attached to your natural teeth with metal clasps or devices called precision attachments. This is shown on the patient's records as P/– or –/P.

In every case, the first appointment will be for impressions. In most cases the second appointment will be for the *bite* stage, during which measurements are taken in the treatment room, so that the lab will know how the patient's jaws relate to each other and can place the centre line of the patient's face. At this point the dentist and patient will decide upon the type, shape and shade of teeth required and inform the lab. The third stage is the *try-in*. By this stage the lab have mounted the selected teeth on to a wax denture so the dentist can re-check the bite and the patient can see how the finished denture will look in their mouth. If all is well at this stage, the denture proceeds to the *fit* stage. If the dentist or patient is unhappy with the wax try-in, alterations will be made and a *re-try* requested. For some partial dentures there is no need for a bite stage, whereas for some metal dentures additional stages will be required.

Table 6.5 Dentures: considerations.

Needs to be considered	
Treatment room	When booking the appointment, consideration should be given to forwarding the impressions to the lab quickly, to prevent deterioration of the impression materials. The number of impressions required will depend upon the type of denture required. The appointments will be relatively short; book all four appointments separated by approximately one week at the beginning of the course of treatment. Each appointment should be booked at a time you can be certain the lab work will be available in the practice. Most practices request the work back from the lab one working day before the patient's appointment.
Patient	The patient should be given a clear idea of how long they will spend in the treatment room on each visit and how many visits they will need. Patients must understand the importance of keeping all four appointments and that if they fail to keep any one appointment the subsequent appointments may be cancelled by the practice. Details of payment requirements should be clarified when booking the appointments. Payment should be collected to ensure the laboratory invoices are always covered and before the denture is fitted.

In some cases dentures will be placed immediately after an extraction to replace a front tooth. This is referred to as immediate restoration (IR). Such dentures proceed from impressions directly to fit. In this case, after impressions have been taken, the patient will require an appointment for extractions (XLA) and fit (Table 6.5).

Emergencies

Every practice will have time set aside for dental emergencies. It is important that the practice provides the receptionist with clear guidelines about what qualifies as an emergency, as often the dentist may not regard what patients consider to be an emergency in the same way.

Although the receptionist will be aware of what the practice considers to be an emergency, patients may try to fool the system by exaggerating symptoms and saying they are in severe pain when they are not. It is advisable to have an emergency checklist on the reception desk and record patients' responses to questions asked. (See Table 6.6.)

Table 6.6 Emergencies: considerations.

Needs to be considered	
Treatment room	The practice policy must outline what qualifies as an emergency, when an appointment should be offered and how much time should be booked for pain management, lost crowns, broken teeth and lost fillings. Preset questions should be asked at the time of booking, to ascertain if the patient suffers from any conditions which may delay treatment being carried out on the emergency visit.
Patient	The patient should be given a clear idea of how long they will be given for an emergency appointment, and that, depending upon the problem, they may need to return for further visits. Care should be taken when working with people who are in pain. The receptionist should show empathy and be supportive, always stressing what you can do rather than what is not possible. Never say anything that might be interpreted as being prescriptive; the receptionist should simply gather and record information for the dentist.

Extractions

Removing teeth is a treatment of last resort, for teeth beyond repair, or when patients cannot afford restorative treatments. Most extractions are straight-forward, although in some cases, when a general dental practitioner has concerns about the patient's general health or when a general anaesthetic is required, extractions are referred to an oral surgeon. When a referral to a specialist is necessary, you will need to inform the patient that they will receive their appointment directly from the specialist. Indicate to them how long you expect it will take for them to receive an appointment and ask them to get in back in touch with you if, after this length of time, they have not received an appointment (Table 6.7).

Fillings

When tooth tissue is damaged or worn, teeth can be restored with filling materials. There are numerous materials in common use for this purpose. Many people have metal fillings. These can be either amalgam (silver) or gold filling restorations. Tooth-coloured composite resin fillings are a popular alternative to traditional metal fillings and look like natural tooth tissue. Composite resin fillings are strong and durable, and make for a very natural-looking smile. Many dentists recommend composite fillings to their patients to avoid the use of mercury-based amalgam. However, the cost of composite

Table 6.7 Extractions: considerations.

Needs to be considered	
Treatment room	Surgical extractions should not be booked in close succession to each other, to allow time for specialist equipment to be sterilised for each patient when successive patients require extractions from the same quadrant of their mouths. The dentist will tell you how much time is required for each individual patient. Additional time may be required for patients to recover and for the dentist to ensure that the bleeding has stopped, in addition to the time required for the actual extraction.
Patient	Inform the patient that for extractions under local anaesthetics it is advisable they eat before attending for their appointment. Ensure that patient is not going to be doing anything strenuous after the procedure and that they will be able to take it easy for the remainder of the day. Ensure that patient is given an after-extraction advice sheet. This will advise that if they are in pain after the extraction they should take what they would normally take for a headache, *as long as it is not aspirin*. They are advised to contact the practice if the pain persists after a few days. Make sure the patient is aware of costs and payment requirements before the extraction takes place.

fillings is considerably greater than the cost of traditional amalgam fillings because the materials are more expensive and more surgery time is required to place them.

The dentist will need to inform reception of the length of time required. In most cases this information will be entered on to the patient's notes before they are presented to the receptionist. An experienced receptionist will know how long individual dentists need to carry out each type of filling restoration. Whenever there is any doubt about the length of time required, check with the prescribing dentist or their nurse before booking the appointment (Table 6.8).

Gingivectomy

This is a surgical procedure for treating gum disorders. A gingivectomy is a periodontal procedure for the surgical removal of excess gum tissue, which has not responded to treatment by conventional means. Some dentists refer this type of gum surgery to a specialist periodontist. It is a minor oral surgery procedure requiring sterile techniques. Patients will require two or three

Table 6.8 Fillings: considerations.

Needs to be considered	
Treatment room	When booking an appointment, consideration should be given to the type of filling being placed, as composite fillings take longer to place than amalgam fillings.
Patient	Tell the patient how long they will be under treatment. This will depend on the filling material being used, as composite fillings take longer to place than amalgam fillings. Explain that their mouth will be numb after the appointment and advise they have a light meal before attending.
	Check that details of all fillings are included in the patient's written treatment estimate.

spaced appointments. The first is for the gingivectomy, the second for a follow-up appointment to remove any stitches and the third a follow-up to monitor the healing process (Table 6.9).

Implants

Crowns, bridges or dentures are not the only options when it comes to replacing missing teeth. For some people, dental implants offer another option. Surgically placed below the gums over a series of appointments, implants fuse to the jawbone and serve as a base for individual replacement teeth, bridges or dentures. Because implants fuse to the jawbone, replacement teeth feel natural.

This is a time-consuming, intensive and high-cost treatment. In some cases patients will be referred for a CT scan to ensure the dentist has a clear view of details of the nerves and sinuses prior to placing the implant or in order to prepare for bone grafting (Table 6.10).

Inlays and onlays

These offer alternative methods of repairing teeth when more than half of the biting surface is damaged. Made of porcelain or gold they are cast to the exact shape of the tooth and bonded to the damaged area of a tooth. An inlay is similar to a filling and lies inside the cusp tips of the tooth; an onlay is a more extensive reconstruction that includes one or more cusps of a tooth (Table 6.11).

Inlays and onlays are applied in two dental visits. At the first visit the old filling, or decay, is removed, and the tooth is prepared for the inlay/onlay. The dentist will then make an impression of the tooth, and send this impression to a dental laboratory. This impression will be used by the laboratory to construct the inlay/onlay. At the second visit the dentist will ensure

Table 6.9 Gingivectomy: considerations.

Considerations	
Surgery needs	Gingivectomy appointments should not be booked in close succession to each other. This is because specialist equipment, which will need to go through rigorous sterilising techniques before it is used on another patient, may be in short supply. Therefore do not book more than one gingivectomy in any session. The nurse will require time before the patient arrives to make the treatment room ready. When booking follow-up appointments, there may be a need to link the appointment with the dentist to one with the hygienist, who will ensure that the patient's home care procedures are adequate to secure the benefits of the treatment.
Patient needs	Tell the patient how long they will be under treatment, and what they can expect afterwards. The patient should be advised how long the procedure will take and to have a light meal before the appointment. They need to understand that their mouth will be numb for some time after the appointment and to avoid hot or hard foods until the gums are healed. Ensure that written consent is gained for treatment to proceed. Make sure the patient leaves with a postoperative advice sheet.

Table 6.10 Implants: considerations.

Needs to be considered	
Treatment room	Implants are advanced surgical procedures requiring the highest standards of cross-infection control and sophisticated equipment. Throughout the procedure two nurses will assist the surgeon. A considerable amount of diagnostic work will take place before the treatment commences, the results of which must be available to the surgeon at each of the appointments.
Patient	Ensure that written consent is gained for treatment to proceed. Give aftercare (post-operative) advice sheet.

Table 6.11 Inlays and onlays: considerations.

Needs to be considered	
Treatment room	When booking appointments for inlays and onlays, consideration should be given to forwarding the impressions to the lab quickly to prevent deterioration. Inlay/onlay preps should not be booked in rapid succession to each other. If the inlay/onlay is being manufactured at the practice, only one visit is required. Otherwise, the 'inlay/onlay fit' appointment should be made for a time when you are sure that the finished inlay/onlay will definitely have been returned from the lab.
Patient	The patient should be given a clear idea of how long they will spend in the treatment room on each visit. They need to be aware that their mouth will be numb for a short while after the appointment and that a temporary filling will be in place after the first appointment until the fit appointment. Details of payment requirements should be clarified when booking the appointments. From a financial point of view the inlay/onlay should be fitted as soon as possible after it is returned from the lab to ensure the patient has paid for it before the lab invoices the practice.

that the inlay/onlay fits properly in the tooth and does not interfere with the bite. Once correctly placed, it is bonded into the tooth with a strong bonding resin and polished until smooth.

Oral surgery

Oral surgery is a broad field that addresses the different problems that can occur within the mouth. Most are related to the teeth, though some problems may involve the jaw or the gums. The most common oral surgery treatments carried out in general dental practice are apicectomies, in which the infected apex of a tooth is treated; biopsies for soft tissue abnormalities; and the surgical removal of impacted teeth.

Ample time must be allowed and suitably trained nursing staff must be available to assist the surgeon in preparing the treatment room for surgical procedures and to support the patient throughout the procedure (Table 6.12).

Orthodontics

This dental specialty concentrates on the alignment of teeth in the jaws. Orthodontic treatment aims to straighten teeth to improve function and make home care easier for the patient. Treatments can span 1–3 years, during which

Table 6.12 Oral surgery: considerations.

Needs to be considered	
Treatment room	Oral surgery requires the use of specialised instruments; these are likely to be in short supply so do not book more than one surgical appointment in any session without checking with the head nurse. In some cases two nurses will be needed in the surgery. All x-rays will need to be available to the dentist at the time of the appointment.
Patient	Ensure that written consent is obtained for treatment to proceed. Give aftercare (postoperative) advice sheet. Patients should be advised to eat a light meal before their appointment. Check that the patient has been given dressings in case they are required and explain what postoperative pain they may experience.

time the patient will need to attend every 3–4 weeks for the dentist to monitor and adjust appliances.

Some orthodontic conditions are treated with removable appliances. These treatments are more likely to be carried out by general dental practitioners (GDPs) whereas, when fixed appliances are required, it is more likely that the patient will be referred to a specialist practitioner.

Many orthodontic patients need teeth to be extracted to make space into which crowded teeth can move, through the use of an orthodontic appliance. When patients are referred to specialists, the specialist will give the GDP instructions for the removal of any teeth deemed necessary. The receptionist will be involved in the correspondence process at this time (Table 6.13).

Ozone
Ozone is a form of oxygen and a natural biocide that effectively kills bacteria. When ozone is applied to the tooth surface it kills the bacteria that cause tooth decay and sterilises the site. After the debris has been removed a filling can replace damaged tooth material. This treatment is not available on the NHS (Table 6.14).

Periodontal treatments
Periodontal disease (also known as periodontal infection, gum disease or pyorrhoea) is an ongoing bacterial infection in the gums and bone which support the teeth. If not treated, this ongoing infection can destroy the bone around the teeth resulting in tooth loss. Seventy five percent of all adult tooth loss is due to periodontal infection. The first appointment booked with the

Table 6.13 Orthodontics: considerations.

Needs to be considered	
Treatment room	Orthodontic patients will require a wide range of treatment and assessment appointments, including the initial ortho assessment, treatment planning, regular check-up assessments, impressions, extractions, fit appliances, and appliance adjustments.
	Visits will be short and fairly frequent, to monitor the progression of the treatment.
Patient	Orthodontic treatment involves moving teeth through bone. This can be an uncomfortable process. Patients need the support of the dental team and a programme of patient education to help them manage their treatment at home. Good oral hygiene is a prerequisite for this treatment and must be maintained throughout.

Table 6.14 Ozone: considerations.

Needs to be considered	
Treatment needs	Ozone treatment appointments usually take longer than regular fillings. Other than the ozone unit, there are no special treatment room needs.
Patient needs	Patients need to understand the importance of using the recommended toothpaste and mouthwash as part of their home care routine.

periodontist will be for an assessment, during which decisions will be made about the type of treatment and its duration and cost. Alongside the surgical aspects of treatment, a patient education programme will take place to enable the patient to understand the causes of the condition and to put preventative measures in place (Table 6.15).

Root canal treatments

When decay penetrates the dental pulp, the tooth and the surrounding area are likely to be very painful. Root canal therapy is treatment for disorders of the dental pulp (the soft tissue at the centre of the tooth that contains nerves and blood vessels). Teeth with abscesses or infected nerves were once removed but now, in 95% of cases, the tooth's pulp can be replaced with a synthetic material and the natural tooth saved through root canal treatment (endodontics).

Table 6.15 Periodontal treatment: considerations.

Needs to be considered	
Treatment room	Periodontal treatments can vary from a simple scale and polish to advanced surgical procedures. Always read the surgery notes to ensure you are booking the correct type of appointment, at a time when the necessary equipment and suitably trained nursing staff are available.
Patient	The patient needs to understand how long each appointment will be and what will happen in the treatment room. Patients should be reminded to have a small meal before attending. Treatment cost and payment terms should be met before treatment commences.

Table 6.16 Root canal treatments: considerations.

Needs to be considered	
Treatment room	In general practice, root canal equipment is often shared between surgeries so do not book more than one treatment per session without checking on the availability of equipment as rigorous cross-infection measures are required after each use. In most cases patients will need a series of appointments spaced by 1–2 weeks.
Patient	Tell the patient how long the appointment needs to be and that their mouth will be numb after the first appointment. Make sure the patient has consented to the costs and payment requirements.

Receptionists in general dental practices need to be aware that root fillings cannot be booked in close succession to each other, in order to ensure that the required equipment is available. In some practices equipment is shared between treatment rooms and requires lengthy cross-infection processes to be completed after each use (Table 6.16).

Scale and polish
Scaling is the removal of calcified deposits from teeth above and below the gum line to maintain gum health. This is coupled with polishing of the fillings and teeth to create smooth surfaces to assist home care. Hygienists are qualified to offer this treatment. A combination of electric scalers and hand-scaling instruments is usually used in dental cleaning.

Table 6.17 Scale and polish: considerations.

Considerations	
Surgery needs	These routine treatments can be booked with dentists, therapists or hygienists. Most hygienists will book 20 minutes for a routine scale-and-polish appointment. When a patient has advanced periodontal disease, an initial series of appointments will be required followed up by 3 monthly scaling appointments to keep the condition under control.
Patient needs	Patients often suffer considerable sensitivity after a scale and need to understand the importance of keeping their mouth free from plaque whilst the soft tissues recover from the treatment. Gum disease is often painless until after scaling, so patients are likely to be concerned by post-operative symptoms unless they are thoroughly prepared for them.

Electrical scalers use a tip that vibrates very fast, and is kept cool by a stream of water. The water is removed from the patient's mouth with suction.

For patients with periodontal (gum) disease, scaling may include removing deposits from the roots of the teeth. This is called root planing. When gum is inflamed, gum pockets become deeper and they lose bone connections inside. The deeper the pockets are, the easier it is for them to trap plaque deposits and worsen the condition of the gum. The periodontal pockets really need to be cleaned up in order to stop further inflammation. Root planing requires the insertion of a hand scaler into the gum pockets to clean away the build-up. This will require a local anaesthetic. The hygienist's role includes educating patients in home care routines (Table 6.17).

Veneers

Veneers (porcelain or plastic) are placed over the front teeth to change the colour or shape of the teeth. They are ideal for teeth that are too small or too big, or have uneven surfaces. Veneers solve such irregularities and create a durable and pleasing smile. Veneers are made either in the lab from porcelain or in the surgery. CEREC is a new high-tech system for manufacturing crowns at the practice whilst the patient is in the dental chair.

In many cases, patients request this cosmetic procedure. In this case the receptionist must first book the patient for an assessment of their suitability for the treatment and to agree the treatment fee with the patient. The second appointment will be to prepare the tooth/teeth. The dentist will explain how much time is required, which depends upon the number of teeth to be prepared and whether they need to be built up with filling materials first. The

Table 6.18 Veneers: considerations.

Needs to be considered	
Treatment room	This routine treatment does not require specialist materials. The dentist will specify the time allocated, depending upon how many teeth are being treated and the condition of any existing fillings in the teeth.
Patient	The patient needs to be aware that the teeth being treated may be sensitive after the prep appointment until the veneers are fitted. For this reason it is important to know how long the lab needs to produce the work, and to book the 'fit' appointment as soon as the lab work returns. All payment terms must be met before the prep appointment can take place.

dentist will take impressions for the lab to prepare the veneers, which will be bonded to the teeth at the third appointment.

Whitening

This is a totally private treatment, requested by patients who want a whiter smile. There are numerous tooth-whitening products on the market, some of which are carried out in the dental chair. Others, termed 'at home' bleaching, are carried out by the patient away from the practice.

The term 'chairside bleaching' is sometimes used to refer to tooth whitening procedures performed by dentists. These usually require more than one

Table 6.19 Whitening: considerations.

Needs to be considered	
Treatment room	Each patient must begin this treatment with an assessment appointment during which the impressions will be taken to make the trays if 'at home' bleaching is to be used. If chairside bleaching is preferred, the patient will need to make a long appointment (in excess of 1 hour) for the treatment.
Patient	Some patients experience sensitivity in their teeth and irritation in their gums through bleaching. Using sensitive toothpaste or reducing the use of the gel can easily remedy this. This treatment is not available on the NHS, so terms of business must be agreed before this private treatment begins.

visit. Each visit may take from 30 minutes to one hour, during which the dentist will apply either a protective gel or a rubber shield to protect the oral soft tissues. A bleaching agent is then applied to the teeth, and a special light used to enhance the action of the agent.

At home bleaching methods are very popular and generally less expensive than chairside bleaching techniques. This requires the patient to attend for an initial assessment appointment. If the dentist considers the patient to be suitable for home bleaching, impressions will be taken so that the lab can produce a plastic tray, like a mouthguard, into which bleaching gel is placed and worn for a prescribed number of hours each day for a couple of weeks. As bleaching will not lighten white fillings, crowns and bridges, these may need replacing.

From the practice's point of view, an efficient appointment book provides varied and interesting work in the treatment rooms whilst ensuring that the practice earns the required hourly income to be profitable.

Chapter 7
Administrative Skills

Administrative systems

Efficient and friendly reception services can be an enormous asset for any dental practice. The fact is that unless reception staff are formally trained to run efficient, consistently effective administrative systems, they are unlikely to understand their importance (other than to avoid conflict with angry patients). They are even less likely to understand the importance of carrying out regular system reviews. In 2003 a survey carried out by the British Dental Receptionists' Association revealed that 70% of receptionists held no formal administrative qualifications. So it is fair to assume that their training has been conducted on a hands-on, trial-and-error basis. Although many patients will see the odd minor mistake as an acceptable human error, continuous and disruptive mistakes are less acceptable and are seen by patients as a reflection of the clinical care provided by the practice. This is a pity because it is seldom the case.

> Formal training will develop a person's knowledge, aptitude and understanding of what makes systems work, how they should be designed to be organised and consistent, and the need for results to be regularly evaluated. Such systems are created with the following considerations in mind:
>
> ■ the results the system should achieve;
> ■ the resources needed to operate the system;
> ■ how the results will be measured;
> ■ legal and ethical requirements;
> ■ the avoidance of duplication.

Even now that many reception systems are computer based, these considerations are still relevant, because although computer systems go a long way towards streamlining information, the old adage of 'rubbish in, rubbish out' still holds true. The capabilities of administrators are therefore as relevant in computerised practices as they are in those that are non-computerised.

The creation of systems, rather than the performing of random tasks, is central to good administration. Systems should be created and recorded on paper to prevent the 'Chinese whispers' effect when new team members are being trained.

When designing systems it is advisable to start by focusing upon what you want to achieve. Every practice will run numerous systems, for example the following.

- *the appointment book*: treatments, recalls, follow-ups for missed appointments, cancellations.
- *accounting systems*: patient payments, sales and purchase ledgers, cash sheets, banking, petty cash, claiming NHS fees.
- *marketing activities*: receiving patient feedback, selling of sundry goods, telephone skills.

The list goes on, and for every activity it is important to meet patients' expectations and create a consistently good impression of the professionalism of all the dental team. Patients should experience systems as:

- smooth running;
- accurate;
- informative;
- caring;
- delivered in a relaxed manner.

For systems to be effective they must be as user-friendly for the administrator as they are for patients. The team should experience administrative systems as being:

- reliable;
- straightforward;
- well organised;
- appropriate.

Ten Dos and Don'ts for Administrators

Do

(1) Do **keep accurate records**. Accurate clinical record keeping skills are taught in dental schools. All too often this principle is not carried over into practice administration. Record keeping systems, which form clear audit paths, are essential. Producing a reception manual and following its procedures in a disciplined way will ensure the quality of your systems and comply with legal requirements.

(2) Do **pay attention to detail**. In a busy reception area you will often be expected to work on more than one task at a time. If the pressure created by working in this way leads you to shortcut systems, you will store up problems for the future. Skimming over the details of tasks

can create extra work in the long term and undermine the professionalism of the practice. *Most importantly, keep your working area tidy. A tidy desk portrays a tidy mind.*

(3)   Do **set and follow procedures**. The best way to create an atmosphere of professionalism within practice administration is to plan and follow proven procedures.

(4)   Do **watch for changing needs**. Because a system is working well at the moment does not mean that it will work well forever. Good systems change and adapt to meet changing needs. This does not mean that systems should be changed on a whim. All changes should be made in consultation with all of the systems users and be well documented.

(5)   Do **measure results**. When you receive patient complaints, you know that you are doing something not to their liking. The fact is that, even when unhappy with the service, many patients will not complain, or at least not to you; however, they will complain to anyone else who will listen, as discussed later in this chapter in the section covering patient complaints. It is also a good idea to listen to patients talking to each other in the waiting room and consider how you can improve your practice administration based upon their comments to each other.

Don't

(6)   Don't **duplicate or over complicate tasks**. It's not a good idea to make practice administration any more complicated than it needs to be. Overcomplicated systems lead to mistakes and omissions. Streamline systems.

(7)   Don't **try to be all things to all people**. It is commendable to do what you can to please patients and colleagues alike. However, you can end up by pleasing nobody if you are shortcutting systems and making changes to please one person at the expense of others. The real skill is to know how flexible you can be without creating situations in which you risk pleasing nobody.

(8)   Don't **run out of stock materials**. Running out of the materials you require to do your job is just bad organisation. Always keep stock at a level that will enable you to work smoothly and professionally.

(9)   Don't **jump from job to job leaving loose ends**. Working on a busy reception will often mean that you need to jump from job to job without finishing any of them. Make sure that you return to all of your loose ends and complete tasks so that they cannot bring about nasty shocks in the future.

(10)   Don't **forget to have fun**. When you are enjoying your work you work better. Attitude is everything. The body language given out will affect the way that others react to you and can increase the pleasure or the pain of being a dental receptionist.

The link between efficient and well trained workforces and business success is undisputed. The problem for many dental practices is that to have well trained staff means sending the receptionist on a training course, which in turn means enduring staff shortages and their resulting chaos. In addition, unless you are near a training centre, there is the cost of lengthy and expensive journeys, added to which many well established staff have severe misgivings about commencing a lengthy course of study.

Patient recalls

Most practices operate a recall system to remind patients that a routine assessment is due. Carried out well the recall system reflects a well organised practice with a caring preventative approach. Running a recall system is primarily a client care measure and should meet the needs of both the practice and the patients whilst maintaining practice cash flow. Recall systems must be designed with care since poorly designed systems will not only fail to produce the desired results but will also place reception staff under increased pressure and annoy patients. An example of this would be the practice that sends out 100 recalls by post on the last Friday of each month. As a result, the last days of each month are pure chaos on the reception desk, putting extreme pressure on reception to find appointments for the patients who can get through on the phone. Others will dial the practice number repeatedly and receive the engaged tone, so will stop trying. As a result, such a practice bears the cost of a system that has exhausted their receptionists and exasperated patients.

Recall systems are designed to maintain the flow of patients through the practice. Some overloaded practices have stopped recalling patients to contain the demand for appointments. When practices are unable to appoint patients to complete their treatments, the results for cash flow can be devastating. Overloaded practices risk failing their patients and run a high risk of failing as businesses.

A popular method of recalling patients is to invite patients to book their appointment for their next routine review on completing a course of treatment. This appointment may be linked to a hygienist appointment, or may be simply a routine review appointment. From an administrative point of view this is the ideal, but there will always be patients who do not wish to book their next appointment so far ahead.

Computerised practices use the database built into their dental software of choice to operate recalls. The leading systems offer two review appointment possibilities. One indicates that the patient has booked it and is aware of it; the other just reserves an appointment for the practice to follow up in due course.

Recall letters can be produced by computer at a pre-set length of time before the appointment, usually about three weeks, and posted out. In some practices, at quiet times receptionists contact patients by telephone or text message to book their review appointment. In some cases this method is used to fill cancellation gaps.

As technology advances, automatic systems for recalling patients and reminding them of existing appointments or informing them that an appointment is available will produce excellent results. These methods are low cost and time efficient. Systems enabling patients to book their own review appointments online are already in use in a few practices. As a result the receptionist's time is freed up from routine tasks, enabling reception to expand its face-to-face care coordination measures.

Recall systems work well for many practices; experience shows that systems that allow patients to make their appointments are the most cost- and time-effective method. The problems arising when practices have too many patients and not enough appointments should be addressed responsibly, protecting the interests of loyal long-term patients who provide the stability for the practice.

Handling patient complaints

When in-house complaints schemes first became mandatory in dental practices in 1996 following the Wilson Report's recommendations, there was considerable consternation. It was feared that the creation of complaints mechanisms would drive up the number of complaints, leading to increased litigation. However, many dental teams now see how valuable well handled complaints can be for the improvement of customer-focused services. By following the structured in-house procedure for dealing with complaints about NHS treatments, most patients' complaints can achieve mutually agreeable outcomes.

This is far preferable to what might otherwise happen. Dental patients unhappy with treatments or services will seek treatment elsewhere in future and/or spread word to their friends and relatives of their perceptions of your practice. This can damage your hard-earned reputation. Worse still, the relationship can break down completely and the patient will go to an outside body with their complaint. So, an efficient, user-friendly system to gather patients' comments and complaints will benefit your practice and meet the professional obligations set out in the GDC's Standards for Dental Professionals.

Preparing to deal with complaints

Each practice must designate a member of the team to respond to patients' feedback about your services. To call this person the complaints officer would be a negative approach and could encourage complaints. A much more rounded approach is to let patients know a named person has been designated to receive their complaints, comments and compliments.

The receptionist or practice manager will often be the first person to be made aware of a complaint. When possible, it is advisable to ask patients to make complaints in writing. In this way you have an accurate record of the complaint in the patient's own words. If the patient is not able or willing to complain in writing, make sure you prepare an accurate, dated and written record of events as soon as possible after the complaint is brought to your attention.

Complaints should be acknowledged by return with a standard letter developed in line with advice from the practice's dental protection society, the PCT or the BDA. In the letter state that an investigation into the complaint will take place and that the complainant will be invited into the practice to discuss the results of the investigation within ten days. A detailed record of all contacts between the patient and practice should be made. Should the in-house complaints procedure fail to resolve the situation, your PCT will require these records.

Once the investigation is complete, a meeting should be set up with the patient to discuss the findings and resolve the situation. A negotiation process should be opened. Any offer of redress should be on the basis that it is a gesture of good will, without the practice admitting liability. In cases when the practice is not at fault, it is important to resolve the complaint at this stage. This is more likely to happen if you can avoid saying or implying:

- the practice is right and the patient is wrong;
- the patient has made a mistake.

If the investigation is unable to find any basis for the complaint, acknowledge the patient's feelings. The outcome of any meetings or discussions with patients should be communicated to them in writing and full details of each complaint, investigation and report should be recorded in a complaints file rather than on the patient's clinical records.

Recording complaints
The following details should be recorded:

- The date of receipt of the complaint.
- How the complaint was received.
- Details of the complaint and the subsequent investigation.
- Notes of telephone conversations and meetings.
- A record of the outcome of the complaint.
- All correspondence relating to the complaint.
- An entry should be made on the patient's records that a complaint has been made.

Over recent years the GDC has produced very good patient information leaflets about their role and how the public can approach them when they have concerns. More recently, they have created a scheme, the Dental Complaints Service, to help resolve complaints from private patients.

Dental Complaints Service (DCS)

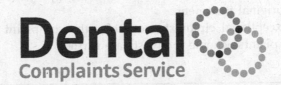

During 2005, legislation was passed empowering the GDC to create the Dental Complaints Service. The service primarily covers complaints from private patients about all aspects of their dental care (treatments and services) and all members of the dental team. The DCS takes dental complaints handling a step further, operating at arm's length from the GDC from its base in Croydon. It is separate from the GDC's fitness to practice procedures.

The scheme provides a service for private patients who are not served by the NHS complaints process. Protocols are in place with the NHS setting the ways in which the DCS handles complaints about mixed private and NHS treatment in order to avoid two organisations trying to resolve the same complaint. This is how the scheme works.

Stage 1 – Helpline information

Whilst the service is aimed at private patients, when anyone has a query or concern about dental care they have received, they will be able to call the telephone helpline. A complaints advisor will then establish what the caller's query is and give them information about their options. The public will also be able to make their enquiries by e-mail or post. Patients will be encouraged to take matters up with the practice in the first instance. In cases where the issues raised appear to have serious implications for the safety of the public, or if it appears that a criminal offence has been committed, callers may be directed to the relevant authorities.

Stage 2 – Complaints resolution service

Where complaints related to NHS treatments have not been resolved at the practice level, patients will be directed to the appropriate NHS organisation. For non-NHS treatments the scheme will act as an intermediary between the patient and the practice. If this does not resolve the issues, the advisor will refer the case to a panel for consideration. Such panels are held locally, with the possibility of regionally based panels being formed depending on the workload.

Stage 3 – The outcome

The panel will be able to make any of the following recommendations:

- Close the case with no further action taken.
- Close the case, making recommendations for future practice.
- Recommend that an apology be made by the dental professional concerned and/or that a refund be paid of treatment costs and/or towards the costs of remedial treatment, where appropriate, limited to the cost of the original treatment.
- In exceptional circumstances, refer the complaint to the Director of the Complaints Scheme to investigate further.

Your role in handling complaints

Never underestimate the importance of a complaint. Be positive about complaints: look upon them as learning experiences. When handling a complaint you should:

- Listen carefully.
- Gather information.
- Understand and acknowledge the complaint.
- Reassure the patient that you care.
- Take written notes where appropriate.
- Show that you understand.
- Tell the patient that you understand how they feel, and that you can appreciate their feelings.
- Refer to dentist or practice manager.
- Get back to the patient as appropriate without undue delay.
- Generally, take steps to avoid reoccurrence.

The desired results when handling complaints

It is easy to feel hurt or offended when a patient complains. It is important to view the complaint as the patient's way of helping you to correct shortfalls in your services, in fact as a constructive way to help you to:

- gain an insight into the way patients view your practice;
- rectify shortfalls;
- see the practice from the patient's point of view.

Never underestimate the value of complaints. By remaining positive and viewing complaints as learning experiences you are able to continually improve your services to patients.

Chapter 8
Patient Payment Plans

Patient payments

The vast majority of receptionists are very clear and enthusiastic about their role in patient care. There is often less clarity about their role as the practice's financial regulator, the person responsible for ensuring that the money owed to the practice for treatments is collected on time, and/or for implementing the practice's policy for collecting patients' fees. Besides collecting fees, receptionists are also responsible for the safe keeping of money until it is banked.

While patients who consistently fail to keep appointments drain practice resources, the worst type of patients are those who attend, have their treatment and leave without paying. At best they create unnecessary work chasing bad debt; at worst they are a threat to the viability of the practice.

Where bad debts have been a problem in the past, the introduction of a clear policy, consistently followed, reduces bad debts dramatically. Before any dental receptionist can excel as a financial regulator, management measures need to be introduced to provide a clear framework for the role, in the form of practice policies. For example, practice policy for collecting patient's payments may say:

> It is our policy to provide patients with a written estimate and treatment plan, which they are required to sign to indicate their acceptance of the treatment plan and payment conditions before any treatment is undertaken. Our policy is that:
>
> - Patients are required to pay at each visit for the treatment carried out.
> - All new patients are required to pay £30.00 in advance at their first appointment.
> - We reserve the right to ask any patient to pay for their treatment in advance.
> - When treatment costs are in excess of £200.00, a 50% deposit is required in advance of booking.
> - No further appointments can be booked for patients with fees outstanding.
> - For cancellations with less than 48 hours notice and for missed appointments it is our policy to charge £10 for every 10 minutes booked. These fees will be classed as an outstanding balance.
> - Fees can be paid by cash, cheque, or credit or debit card.
> - Unpaid fees will be subject to a 2% administration charge, and possible court action for collection.

Recording patients' payments

Keeping accurate and reliable financial records not only makes good business sense, it also meets the practice's legal obligations. Practices must ensure that their procedures for recording patients' payments comply with tax and company law; the Inland Revenue requires financial records to be accurate and transparent. Computerised practices using modern dental software packages benefit greatly from the built-in accountancy packages. With a touch of a button, they are able to reconcile fees earned in the treatment rooms with moneys banked. Receptionists benefit too as they are less likely to be suspected of dishonesty, as can be the case when ill-defined or slapdash procedures lead to suspicion and mistrust. If money were to go missing, with robust accounting systems it is easy to pin down the source of problems. Stringent money-handling procedures produce audit trails and protect staff from the stigma of unfounded suspicion and the practice from theft.

Taking patients' payments

The receptionist's role in maintaining cash flow is key to financial success. When patients arrive at the practice, the receptionist should check the status of their account and take action, in line with practice policy, to keep all accounts up to date, avoiding the need to recover bad debts.

Before treatment begins, patients must be given a treatment plan and a written estimate of costs, which they are required to sign to indicate their acceptance. Most practices offer a range of payment methods such as cash, cheque, debit card or credit card. In some cases practices also offer in-house loyalty or corporate care plans, and with the help of finance companies are increasingly making interest-free credit available.

For each payment method offered, the practice should have clear procedures in place developed in response to the recognised costs and benefits linked to the payment method.

Payment option: cash

Benefits
- No percentage taken by third party.
- Funds available as soon as paid into the bank.

Costs
- Risks of holding cash in the practice.
- Risks linked to transporting large sums of cash to the bank.
- Consumer credit regulations on taking large sums in cash must be observed.

When taking patients' payments in cash the following measures should be observed:

- Always count any change due into the patient's hand, to avoid accidental errors and so that there is mutual agreement that the right change has been given.
- Never put the patient's money into the till until they have accepted their change.
- When the patient has accepted their change, place money into the till immediately.
- Secure the till drawer closed.
- Record details of payment.
- Issue a receipt.

Payment option: cheque

Benefits
- No percentage taken by third party.
- Cheques can only be paid into the payee's bank account.

Costs
- It takes days for cheques to clear.
- Patients could stop their cheques.
- Asking for cheque guarantee card number, which must be written on the back of the cheque by the receptionist and not the patient, might be construed as mistrust of the patient.

When patients' payments are made by cheque, the receptionist should ensure that:

- The cheque is correctly dated.
- The cheque is signed.
- It is made out for the right amount.
- It has words and figures that match.
- It is made payable to the correct name.
- It is supported by a bankers card: write the number and expiry date on the back of the cheque.

When satisfied that the cheque is valid:

- Enter details on to computer, checking all figures.
- Issue a receipt to patient.
- Place cheque in the till.

Payment option: credit or debit card

Debit card

Benefit
- Funds appear in the practice account in the same way as a cheque, but patient cannot stop the debit.

- Pin numbers make payments more secure.
- No need to transport money to the bank: payment by electronic transfer.

Costs
- A small fixed fee is charged by bank for administration.

Credit card

Benefits
- No need to transport money to the bank: payment by electronic transfer.

Costs
- A percentage of the total amount is charged by the bank for administration.
- Risk of fraud – time spent by staff checking end-of-month statements.

When taking payment by debit/credit card the receptionist should:

- Check expiry date on card.
- Place card firmly in the pin code machine.
- Press sale button and wait for machine prompts.
- Machine will ask you to enter amount of sale; always double-check figures before pressing enter.
- Machine will prompt patient to enter pin number.
- If there is a problem with the chip on the card, then machine will issue sheet for signature. In this case, ask patient to check and sign slip whilst you remove card and check that signature matches.
- Top copy of the slip is kept by the practice, and the pink copy underneath is handed back to the patient with their card.
- Enter details on to the computer, checking all figures.
- Issue receipt to patient.
- Place slip in the till.

Payment option: loyalty scheme
Patients make monthly payments into the scheme for their routine care by direct debit, spreading the cost of their basic dental care. These schemes guarantee an income to the practice whether or not patients attend. Such schemes aim to ensure patients attend regularly, as they have already paid for their routine visits.

Benefits
- Regular income for the practice.
- Allows patients to spread payments for routine care.
- Entitles patients to discounted treatment fees.
- Many schemes include accident insurance.

Costs

- Some patients object to making additional payments when treatment is required.
- The practice needs to record monthly payments on patients' records.

Payment option: loan

Under the Consumer Credit Act it is an offence to collect payments in more than six instalments unless you have a consumer credit licence issued by the Office of Fair Trading. When treatment fees are extensive, some patients prefer to apply for finance to meet the charges. A number of companies now offer interest-free loans to dental patients. Practices need to register to access these services and must hold a consumer credit licence.

Benefits

- The practice receives payment immediately the loan is agreed.
- The credit company takes the risk if the patient defaults on the loan.

Costs

- Inconvenience of filling in forms and making telephone calls.
- The loan is free to the patient but the practice pays a fee.
- The cost of the consumer credit licence.

When no payment is made and there is a balance outstanding

In these circumstances the receptionist should:

- Give the patient an up-to-date statement of their account.
- If, after payment options have been reiterated, there is still no solution, the situation should be referred to the practice manager or dentist.

Treatment costs, especially for cosmetic treatments, can be considerable. We have an absolute duty to be clear with patients about treatment costs and payment requirements.

Security arrangements for cash on practice premises

Any business taking large amounts of cash has a responsibility to make adequate arrangements to protect staff from robbery. Under Health and Safety at Work law (MHSWR), employers are required to assess risks to staff and patients, and ensure action is taken in a timely manner to reduce the risk of harm, as shown in Table 8.1. Practices must identify ways in which employees are placed at risk from work procedures. When large sums of money accumulate in reception, the receptionist faces the threat of robbery. Many practices have not yet recognised the dangers linked to handling large sums of money in a public area and have yet to instigate security measures. In some cases, receptionists place themselves at risk by reconciling the day's takings on the reception desk in front of a waiting room full of people.

Table 8.1 Risk assessment for money on premises.

Hazard	Risk	Who is at risk	Risk management measures
Holding money in the reception area	Being viewed by potential thieves as a soft target for robbery	Reception staff and patients in the waiting room	Limitation of amount of cash held on the desk, by periodically putting moneys into a safe away from reception
Carrying cash to the bank to be paid into the practice account	Being viewed by potential thieves as a soft target for robbery	Person taking money to the bank	Payments into the bank have to be made so this risk cannot be eliminated, but to minimise it go to the bank in twos at various times of day and by various routes
Cashing-up	Reconciling takings at reception with patients in the adjoining patient lounge	Reception staff	End-of-day reconciling should not be commenced until the front door is locked
The perception there are large sums of cash on the premises	Having or being thought to have large sums of cash on the premises	All team members and the practice bank balance	Insurance cover states that no more than £500 should be on the premises overnight, and that it must be locked away. The practice alarm must be activated whenever the premises are vacated. To minimise risks, moneys must be banked daily

As credit cards and cheques become the preferred method of payment, the cash taken in practices is continually reducing. This should reduce the risk. In reality, however, when potential thieves believe there are large amounts of money on the premises, staff remain vulnerable to the threat of robbery.

Informing patients of fees due

A friendly assertive approach works best where payment requests are concerned. Communication is the cornerstone of effective fee collection. Written estimates are the payment contract between the patient and the practice. Even when patients are in breach of contract, avoid taking a confrontational stance, especially in public areas of the practice; instead offer a private talk with the practice manager. Payments not collected become bad debts, which must be carefully monitored and pursued in an efficient and professional manner. Ideally there should be no bad debts, but in reality this is not always achievable.

Procedure for following up overdue accounts

When a patient does not clear their account at the end of their appointment, the account becomes overdue and a *'now due'* letter should be issued. This informs the patient that there is a fee due, states the balance of the account and gives a date by which payment is to be made. At this point, reiterate the methods of payment accepted, and close the letter saying that accounts paid on time help to keep costs down for everyone, and requesting their prompt action in this matter.

After 7 days an *'account reminder'* can be sent to the patient, clarifying the amount outstanding and requesting payment within 7 days. If, after those 7 days have elapsed, the account still remains unpaid, a second, more strongly worded reminder can be sent.

After a further 7 days, if the account still is unpaid, then the final account letter can be sent. This letter informs the patient that if payment is not received within 14 days further action will be taken.

After 7 days, if the account is still unpaid, then a *'notice before proceedings'* form should be completed and sent to the patient, informing them that, unless payment is received by a given date, then immediate proceedings for recovery of the debt may be taken without further notice. It also gives full details of the outstanding account.

If payment has not been received after a further 7 days, a decision is required as to whether to forward details to the debt collection agency or the small claims court. A major factor in this decision will be the size of the outstanding account. Debt collection agencies take a percentage of debts recovered, whereas the court system is easy to use and all court fees are reclaimed from the debtor if judgement is awarded in your favour. However, success in court depends upon the practice being able to provide accurate, detailed evidence of the history of the debt and all measures taken for its recovery. There are issues of confidentiality and data protection that must be observed when following up debts. The guidelines set out by the BDA and contained in their advice sheets should always be followed. Advice can be taken from the local health authority when setting up a bad debt recovery process.

NHS and private care options

Since the early 1990s the vast majority of dental practitioners have reduced or even stopped offering NHS dental services to their patients. For most practitioners this decision was based on two factors. One was the desire to regain clinical freedom eroded by legislative changes as well as by amendments to NHS regulations, and the second was to safeguard the financial security of their businesses.

Whilst the Government insists it is committed to making NHS treatment available to everyone, the reality is different. Most dental patients are unable to register with a local NHS dentist because few provide NHS treatment and when they do it is for certain categories, such as children or patients on benefits who are exempt from fees. Where patients are able to access NHS care, they pay a contribution towards the fees for their treatment. Unlike the rest of the NHS, where services are free at the point of delivery, dental treatments provided in practice incur charges.

This chapter explores the merits and drawbacks of NHS and private treatment options for dentists and their patients.

NHS dental care: the background

In the past, dentists were paid for each item of treatment completed. The practice claimed a fee per item of service provided. For patients exempt from NHS dental fees, the full treatment charges were met by the NHS. Non-exempt patients were required to pay 80% of the NHS fees, with the remainder of the fee, plus a small monthly capitation payment for every NHS patient on the practice's list, being paid by the NHS. From the 1990s many dentists struggled to provide acceptable levels of patient care under the scheme as the fees paid by the NHS were considered to be too low. Meanwhile the requirements made of dentists were increasing, particularly with the introduction of new cross-infection control measures. This was when the exodus from the NHS began. Dentists had the freedom to make this decision because they were not NHS employees. Principals own their own practices and many associates work for practice owners under a self-employed contract.

Personal Dental Service (PDS)

Over many years there have been a series of attempts to reform the way in which dentistry is provided under the NHS. Under the terms of the NHS (Primary Care Act) 1987, a series of pilot schemes were set up in order to discover new ways for dentists and NHS Trusts to work in conjunction with health commissioners to develop ways of delivering NHS dentistry in future.

As part of the Government's commitment to modernise the NHS and to provide accessible, convenient services to patients, PDS pilot schemes were introduced in 1998 to raise levels of patient care and improve oral health locally. These early pilots included a number of general dental practitioners moving into PDS arrangements. Later waves of PDS pilots concentrated on a Trust-led salaried approach and the introduction of Dental Access Centres, most of which were located in areas with poor oral health. In 2002, when the pilots were completed and evaluated, the Chief Dental Officer for England issued a report of their findings entitled 'NHS Dentistry Options for Change'. Under the terms of PDS, Primary Care Trusts (PCTs) had commissioned NHS dental services from local dental practices in line with the Health and Social Care (Community Health and Standards) Act 2003 and the needs of the local population. From 1 October 2005 PCTs became responsible for providing NHS dental services. In some cases they have contracted with NHS primary care dentists and where necessary they provide some services themselves. Practices transferred into PDS over a two-year period, supported by a dedicated support team at the Dental Practice Board in Eastbourne. Known as the PCT Liaison Team, their role was to:

- Be a point of contact and information for PCTs or practices.
- Provide general advice to PCTs regarding PDS. This includes, for example, the handling of patient charge revenue and superannuation contributions.
- Advise PCTs on the practical steps in transferring a practice into PDS.
- Advise practices on the procedures associated with opening a new PDS contract.

Practices do not make the decision to leave the NHS lightly; such decisions are made after much soul searching and consideration of patients' best interests and the viability of the practice. Nevertheless, many patients had mixed feelings about their dentist's withdrawal from the NHS. The merits and drawbacks of NHS care from the patients' perspectives are explored in Table 8.2 and from the practice point of view in Table 8.3.

Non-NHS dental care – the background
Even dental practices in economically deprived areas provide some treatments not available on the NHS on a private or independent basis, mixing NHS and private care within the same treatment plan to provide the most appropriate care for their patients' needs. In more affluent areas it is common to find that it is only children and exempt patients who are offered NHS treatment. With the spectre of PDS looming on the horizon, large numbers of practices in more affluent areas withdrew from the NHS completely and offered treatment on private, pay-as-you-go, independent or private capitation terms only.

Private capitation schemes
There are numerous private capitation schemes available. Here is an outline of some the best known schemes.

Practice Plan
Practice Plan is a very popular provider of independent, practice-branded payment schemes. Patients make a monthly payment by direct debit, which entitles them to specific assessments and preventative treatments plus discounts on regular treatment fees when curative treatments are prescribed. The scheme aims to provide the practice with:

Table 8.2 Merits and drawbacks of NHS care from the patient's perspective.

Merits	Drawbacks
A written estimate and treatment plan is provided, detailing the NHS and private treatment you have agreed to	Not all patients can find a dentist willing to provide NHS dental treatment
Practices are required to produce a practice information leaflet (PIL) outlining their services and terms of business	When you can find a NHS dentist, you may well have to wait months for treatment
Dentists are contracted to provide all necessary treatment to secure and maintain oral health	Cosmetic care options are not available on the NHS
Dentists are required to provide free repair and replacements for treatments that fail within a year	Fee paying patients pay towards their treatment costs
Dentists are required to reserve appointments to provide advice and, where necessary, treatment in an emergency	Dentists need the NHS's prior approval to provide certain treatments
Treatment charges are set by the Department of Health. Exempt patients receive care free of charge	
There is a maximum charge per course of treatment	
Formal procedures for addressing complaints from patients must be in place	

- a regular monthly income;
- protected hourly rates;
- flexible fee levels;
- clinical freedom.

'Practice Plan provides a proven system that earns you a regular income, protects your hourly rate for examinations and hygiene as well as treatment, retains your practice identity and is one in which you, your staff and your patients can believe.' Taken from the Practice Plan's website, www.practiceplan.co.uk.

Denplan

Denplan was launched in 1986 to offer patients a new way to fund non-NHS dental care and provide support services to practices. Patients paid a set amount per month, defined by their past dental status, for dental treatment prescribed by their dentist. It is the first and best known of the schemes in the UK, which have helped patients convert to private care. The company is part

Table 8.3 Merits and drawbacks of NHS care from the practice's perspective.

Merits	Drawbacks
Practices receive regular income from contract	NHS regulations restrict clinical freedom
Maintaining an NHS income enables the practice to continue to receive NHS benefits such as reimbursement of non-domestic rates and maternity payments	Prior approval is required for some treatments
	The NHS sets prices for NHS treatments
NHS occasional treatments can be provided to non-registered patients	Overloaded appointment books mean long waiting times for treatment on the NHS and restrict cash flow
The NHS makes payment for exempt patients' treatments	NHS administration is time consuming
	NHS fees for some treatments do not meet the cost of providing that treatment

of the PPP healthcare group, which is a member of the Global AXA Group. They have an 80% share of the market in independent capitation plans. Around a third of the UK dental profession are members of Denplan and there are nearly one million Denplan-registered patients.

With the introduction of the Denplan Excel Accreditation programme, Denplan helps dentists provide benchmarks in dental care. Denplan practices can either set their own fee levels within up to five pricing bands, or by offering patients the Denplan Essentials plan they are able to provide a basic level of dental care required to monitor the oral health of the patient for a minimal monthly fee. This level of cover usually includes:

■ routine periodic examinations as agreed by the dentist;
■ scaling and polishing as agreed by the dentist;
■ x-rays as agreed by the dentist;
■ A&E cover (same as Denplan Care).

When patients require additional treatments, they are entitled to a discount on private treatment fees.

Dental Payment Administration Services (DPAS)

Another popular scheme, DPAS, handles the administration for dentists wishing to offer an independent, practice-branded payment plan. The scheme recognises that truly independent dental practices want to control their earning power, on either a capitation or private fee per item basis or through a mix of both. DPAS can provide bespoke administration services. Its services are supplemented by international accident and emergency insurance cover and a 24-hour helpline.

DPAS offers practices the benefit of expertise in providing dental administration services and advice from dentists who have led the way in applying the principles of continuing care in their own practices.

Dental Maintenance Plan (DMP)

DMP is a 'hands on' private dental plan launched to provide flexible payment plans for private patients, tailored to the individual requirements of the dentist/practice. Through an association with several well respected organisations, DMP provides a complete development programme for dental practices which includes:

- business management;
- financial management, including correct hourly rate setting and pricing your services to patients on the scheme;
- Human resource training on site or through distance learning;
- CPD advice.

'We are a company owned and run by established, well-known dentists. We are dentists working for dentists and patients, in promoting high quality private practice with colleagues interested in Continuous Professional Development.'

The merits and drawbacks of non-NHS care from the patient's perspective are explored in Table 8.4 and the point of view of dental practices is explored in Table 8.5.

From the patient's point of view, many of the drawbacks linked to private dental care are financial. For this reason an increasing number of practices offer patients the opportunity to access loans from financiers to pay for their treatments. The cost of dental care is a major concern for many people in the UK, particularly retired people exempted from other NHS charges such as prescription fees. In general, the number of people not able to afford regular dental care can only rise in direct ratio to the increased cost of care. This is a real concern for dental professionals with a vocation to enable patients to secure dental health gains.

Sales of dental goods

Over recent years, patients have come to expect to be able to buy dental products in the reception area of their chosen dental practice. This being the case, the provision of dental products for sale in practices can be viewed as a service to patients. Nevertheless there are a number of factors that reception should be aware of, to ensure that the interests of both the practice and patients are served when selling dental goods to patients.

Table 8.4 Merits and drawbacks of non-NHS care from the patient's perspective.

Merits	Drawbacks
Offers cosmetic treatments not available on the NHS	Private fees are higher than NHS fees and vary between dentists
In many cases appointments are more readily available	The cost of superior laboratory processes for lab work is transferred to the patient
Crown/bridge treatments normally completed within a week	Treatment costs are determined by the running costs of the practice
Appointments are usually longer to give the dentist time to spend with the patient	
A greater choice of appointment times, some available out of surgery hours	
Value for money	
Able to demand a higher standard of service, information and environment	

Table 8.5 Merits and drawbacks of non-NHS care from the practice's perspective.

Merits	Drawbacks
The practice can set their own prices to cover running expenses	Patients are more demanding
Able to offer patients treatment not available on the NHS	Patients require a greater selection of appointment times
It is more satisfying to work without the pressures of the NHS	Longer appointment times are required
Substantial decrease in workload and stress	Staff expect higher salaries in private practice
Practice equipment can be upgraded	Loss of NHS benefits if completely a private practice
Less administration	Some patients simply cannot afford treatment fees and their dental health is compromised
The practice team can concentrate on patients' clinical and personal needs	

The professional status of dentists means that they have a duty of care to ensure, as far as possible, that the products they sell to their patients are scientifically proven to be safe and suitable. This places a responsibility upon the dentist to research all products they endorse by selling and to ensure that sufficient information is passed on to patients at the point of sale to enable them to make an informed choice to buy.

How can patients make the right choices when selecting products? We can be sure patients are purchasing products suited to their dental needs by offering products and supporting them to make informed choices. Some patients will need specialist home care products, such as orthodontic brushes, which are not always available in supermarkets. For these patients it is important that practices help their patients by making products available.

By offering products for sale, you are ensuring that the products you recommend are readily available and thereby preventing patients from opting for easily obtainable, familiar or cheaper and less effective substitutes. The range of dental home care products available in the average supermarket is vast. As dental practices are businesses, the profits from the sale of goods are a consideration. Sales levels and profit margins vary vastly from practice to practice. At the very least it is important to cover the costs of purchasing the goods, product promotions, displays and stock management. These tasks are often the responsibility of the reception team or care coordinator. To perform these tasks well requires the development of a range of retail skills as follows.

Purchasing

This means identifying trends and fashions so that you can buy in goods to interest the consumers. It is a good idea to keep an eye open for the big company advertising campaigns in the media so that you can benefit from their advertising expenditure, offering goods that have already been heavily sold to patients by the manufacturer. You should also keep records of what sells and when, so that you can prepare for any seasonal trends. Storage space can be a problem in some practices, and it is important to make sure products are suitably stored.

Product promotion

You need to let patients know about the range of products you sell and make them easy for patients to buy. It is a good idea to ask patients if they would like any information on the products and if they would like to buy. This means that reception needs to be well informed about the features and benefits of products. Yes, even the toothbrushes.

Displays

Presentation is very important. Do not be tempted to put all of your stock on display; rather, make an eye-catching display, showing each product clearly marked with its price. This will ensure that you do not lose products through pilfering, whilst giving a professional feel to your sales effort. The days are gone when you could simply have a mug stuffed with toothbrushes for sale on the reception desk.

The receptionist plays just as important a role as any of the other members of the dental team. With the knowledge that is at hand the receptionist very often answers patients' queries either face to face or by telephone. These can range from which toothbrush is best for a young child, or for a patient undergoing orthodontic treatment, to whether fluoride or non-fluoride toothpaste is best. There are of course the more serious queries. For example, a patient has discovered a lump or rough patch in their mouth and wonders whether or not to make an appointment with their dentist. The receptionist who has at hand the current dental health information can advise the patient in such a way as not to cause alarm and at the same time ensure that the patient receives prompt and professional care.

Chapter 9
Computers in Dentistry

Using computers for dental administration

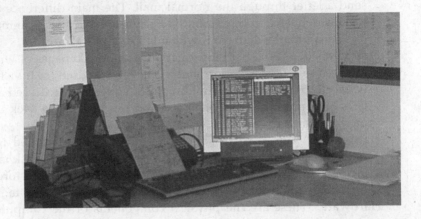

Like it or not, computers impact upon every aspect of modern life. From the kitchen to the workplace, computers make life easier for us. Computerisation in dentistry began in the larger institutions during the 1960s and gathered speed over the past 15 years when practices were offered incentives to computerise their clinical and management systems. This section aims to demystify computer technology, and provide some simple guidelines to help you get the best from your computer.

All computers work by performing five basic operations. Competence in using computer technology begins with an understanding of these functions:

Inputting Entering information into a computer system.
Storing Saving inputted information in a place where it can be used and retrieved.
Processing Using computer programs to convert information into the required format.
Controlling Directing the manner and the order in which operations are performed.

Outputting Accessing collated information created from the raw data inputted.

Computer terminology

Back-ups To safeguard information it is essential to back up frequently. This means duplicating computer data so that a copy can be kept in a separate building away from the main database. Back-ups can be stored on pen drives, zip drives, CDs, floppy disks or tapes.

Disks Hard disks, CDs and floppy disks are used to store information.

Electronic data interchange Some computer systems are certificated by the DPB to transmit claims for NHS treatments electronically.

E-mail E-mail is a way of sending mail and communications through an internet connection to another user, in much the same way as you would send a letter through the normal mail. The main difference is that it is usually delivered within minutes. Each user has a specific e-mail address, e.g. anna@sparkledent.com, which is like a postal address.

Floppy disks These hold information: around 300 pages of writing. They are used to safeguard information. They can be used for transferring data between computers or for holding information only required at intervals. CDs hold much more information and can be used to back up the data on your hard drive.

Hard disks This is part of the computer hardware located in the computer's casing or separately. The capacity of your hard disk is one of the factors that govern the programs that your computer can store. The hard disk holds the software programs and the main system data.

Hardware These are the physical components of the computer, e.g. the circuits, keyboard, mouse, disk drives and printer.

Internet The internet is the name given to a worldwide source of information that is held on computers across the world. You access the internet through a phone line and internet service provider (ISP). Millions of computers around the world offer information for other web users to access through the internet.

Modems PCs in different locations can share information through a telephone line using a modem. Treatment details are sent to the Dental Practice Board through modems using the Electronic Data Interchange (EDI) System.

PC Personal computer. All the data is stored in the hard drive of the PC, or, in the case of a network the data is stored at a central server.

Software The programs that are chosen to enable the computer to perform the tasks required. This will consist of a basic operating system, e.g. Windows, plus the specialist software you install to perform specific tasks.

Viruses There are tens of thousands of computer viruses; some are able to destroy all of the information in your computer. Viruses are transferred from PC to PC through floppy disks, internet, email and pirated software. Never use disks in your system with an unknown history or without checking them for viruses. Always use an up-to-date virus guard in your starting-up procedure (booting up).

Computer security measures

Computer users need to be aware of the importance of applying the security measures shown in Table 9.1 for computer security, Table 9.2 for preventing viruses, and Tables 9.3 and 9.4 for safeguarding information.

Computers and the law

The Government and the EEC are responsible for safeguarding the rights of the public and are continuously introducing new laws to protect individuals

Table 9.1 Security.

Do	Don't
Site equipment away from prying eyes	Trail cables
Secure the building when empty	Place a computer next to a radiator, water pipes and other sources of heat and dampness
Keep the computer keys in a safe place	
Get crime prevention advice	Leave any pieces of portable equipment where a thief can steal them

Table 9.2 Defending against viruses.

Do	Don't
Check every disk before inserting into your computer	Use non-standard software
Ensure that your virus checker is up to date	Download unauthorised information from the internet

Table 9.3 Preventing disaster.

Do	Don't
Keep a master copy of your software	Misuse floppy disks
Back up data regularly	Leave disks next to your computer
Weed out extinct documents	

Table 9.4 Safeguarding information.

Do	Don't
Be discreet with data at all times	Divulge any information without authority
Site equipment away from prying eyes	
Keep passwords private and change them	Leave disks, tapes, printouts and faxes lying about
Clear the screen after use	Start using new software before you know how to use it
	Leave the computer logged on when you leave the room

from the misuse of computer technology; here are some of the laws currently in place.

Data protection

Anyone holding information relating to other individuals must comply with the Data Protection Act 1998. The aim of the Act is to protect individuals from the misuse of information held about them. The Act sets down guidelines for the usage, accuracy and storage of data. It requires data holders to re-register every year with the Data Protection Registrar, stating the type of data to be held and how it will be used.

Under the terms of the Act, individuals have the right of access to information held about them. Applications to see a copy of any information held relating to them must be made in writing. When an application for disclosure of information is received:

- A charge of up to £10 can be made for providing the information. This should be explained to the applicant on receipt of their request.
- A response to an access request must be made within 40 days of receipt.
- If information is held, you must supply a copy.
- Information may be withheld if it identifies other individuals outside the practice or if revealing it would risk damaging the patient's health.
- Before disclosing information you must confirm the applicant's identity with a formally witnessed signature supported by photographic proof of identity from a passport or driving licence. Under the Data Protection Act there are heavy fines and penalties for the misuse of information covered by the Act.

Health and safety

Health and safety legislation relevant to computer users was defined in legislation in an extension to existing health and safety law introduced on

1 January 1993 as the Health and Safety (Display Screen Equipment) Regulations. In many ways the 1993 regulations are in line with other health and safety regulations for electrical equipment. In addition they consider workstation comfort and the effect for the operator of spending long periods of time in front of a monitor.

To safeguard computer workers' well-being employers must:

- Carry out a risk assessment and take steps to remedy any hazards identified.
- Ensure workstations meet minimum standards.
- Plan work to allow for changes in workers' activities.
- On request arrange sight tests for significant users.
- Provide health and safety training.

To safeguard your well-being when working at a computer you should:

- Adjust your chair so that you find the most comfortable position for your work. Your forearms should be approximately horizontal and your eyes at the same height as the top of the VDU screen.
- Make sure there is enough space underneath your desk to move your legs freely. Don't sit in the same position for long periods. Change your posture as often as is practicable.
- Adjust your keyboard and screen to get a good keying-in position.
- Make sure you have enough workspace.
- Arrange the screen so that bright lights are not reflected in the screen.
- Make sure that the characters on your screen are in sharp focus.
- Keep the screen free from dirt, grime or finger marks, and use the brightness control on the screen to suit the lighting conditions in the room.

Copyright, Designs and Patents Act 1988

Most computer software is subject to restrictions on its use and cannot be copied, modified, disseminated or used without appropriate permissions from the copyright holder. This means you cannot use software unless you have an agreement with the authorised supplier and must not borrow disks or copy programs.

Computer Misuse Act 1990

Under this Act unauthorised access to computer systems (hacking) and the introduction of viruses is an offence.

Access to Health Records Act 1990

Running parallel to Data Protection law, which applies to records of living patients, this Act extends to cover rights of deceased patients.

As specialised dental software becomes more and more sophisticated, the development of computer skills within dental teams is set to expand, offering opportunities to predict and gain in-depth understanding of trends impacting on the success of the practice.

Use of Microsoft programs

Now that computers are an integral part of most dental practices, dental teams need to develop a range of computer skills to ensure they maximise the benefits of this technology. The potential benefits of computerisation go beyond the appointment book and patients' records to include new ways to communicate with patients and within the team. Computerised communications not only look professional but they also save time. With Microsoft programs, even the novice can create professional-looking documents.

Microsoft Word

Microsoft Word is fundamentally a computerised typewriter. However, once you become familiar with the program you will be able to do much more. Microsoft Word, when first opened, presents the user with a blank screen. Around the top and bottom of the screen are icons that help you create documents easily. The screen is self-explanatory with menu bars at the top of the screen (File, Edit, View, etc.). If you hover the mouse over the icons arranged at the top and bottom of the screen without clicking on them, a description of what they do will appear. This is helpful when you are learning how to use the program.

As many of the documents you send to patients will be standardised, such as missed appointment letters, appointment reminders or welcome packs, even when performing tasks not integrated into the dental software package of choice you will be able to use a Microsoft Word program to mail merge or you could simply 'top and tail' existing documents. To open an existing word file:

(1) Open Microsoft Word by clicking on the Word icon on the desktop.
(2) Click 'File' (at the top left of the screen) and a drop-down menu will appear.
(3) Click 'Open'.
(4) Once you have clicked on 'Open', you can browse the files saved on the computer and open the particular document you require by clicking on it.

If the document you require was one of the last four files used in Microsoft Word, you will find it listed in the File Menu (the drop-down menu that appears when you click on 'File'). Once the file is open you are able to amend the document.

The toolbar at the top of the screen has little icons that are shortcuts to certain procedures.

Saving a document

The icon for saving on the Toolbar is a picture of a disk. Be careful with this option as it is only 'Save' and not 'Save as' and this could mean that you overwrite important information. Saving documents regularly is an important precaution, to stop work being lost due to computer failure. There are two ways to 'Save' in Microsoft Word:

■ Click on the save icon on the top toolbar. Any amendments to the file will be saved. This will *overwrite* the original document.

■ Use 'Save As' when you do not want to overwrite the original document. Click on 'File'. Click on 'Save as' from the dropdown menu. Select a name for the file to be saved under. 'Save as' allows the document to be saved in a new name, and the original document is not overwritten.

Microsoft Word will automatically create a file name which is taken from the first few words in the document. Changing this file name is easy: click and delete the letters, then type in the desired file name. When closing the program, if you have not saved the changes to your document, Microsoft Word will remind you that you have not saved; this prevents you from losing information.

Printing a document

When you have finished modifying a document and you are ready to print, Microsoft Word makes this task easy. There are two ways to print a document:

■ Click on the toolbar icon for printing. This is a picture of a printer on the top toolbar; simply click on this option and one copy of the document will be printed.

■ Click on 'File'. Click on 'Print'. Under the number of copies, simply type in the amount of copies you require. Click 'OK'. Once you have clicked OK the document will start to print.

Throughout the UK there are colleges offering basic computer training such as CLAIT at no charge to the student. The best way to locate a course near you is through Learndirect, whose number will be in your local telephone directory.

E-mails and messaging

Clearly defined systems for routine communication between colleagues enable each person to produce their best work. By its nature teamwork requires the free and frequent exchange of information and ideas between colleagues. Irrespective of where you work in the practice, communication channels are needed to facilitate information sharing with colleagues in other areas of the practice as easily as if you were both in the same room.

Before the introduction of computerised communication systems, most practices relied on intercom systems to broadcast the arrival of patients to the treatment rooms. Unfortunately, this communication system compromises confidentiality as messages sent to the treatment rooms can be clearly audible to everyone in the treatment room and reception areas.

Now, in computerised practices, teams can communicate with each other throughout the day without having to broadcast the information across the practice. As patients arrive, a message is 'clicked' through from the reception to treatment rooms, using a function of their software of choice. For other information, the use of e-mail and instant messaging means every member of the team can be kept up to date about events as they occur, without distracting them from their work.

Electronic mail (e-mail) is a fast and direct way to contact outside suppliers, such as labs and materials suppliers. They are also a convenient way to forward any referrals to specialists, leaving a clear audit trail that enables you to hold permanent records of the correspondence. Increasingly, patients prefer to be contacted by the practice by e-mail, which is a cost-effective way to handle recalls and routine communications.

Instant messaging is a useful and popular way to share non-standard information with others in the practice. Working in real time, with instant messaging two-way discussions can take place through the computer without either party needing to exit other programs in use.

Using electronic mail

E-mails are sent from computer to computer via the internet. Once connected to the internet, e-mail accounts can be set up free of charge, either through your internet service provider (ISP) or with companies such as Yahoo and Hotmail, which allow you to access your e-mails on any computer.

To send e-mails, you need to know the e-mail address of the intended recipient. All e-mail addresses include the '@' symbol, and a specific ending such as .com, .co.uk, etc. A common mistake made by people new to e-mailing is to confuse website addresses and e-mail addresses. Website addresses always begin with 'www.' and e-mail addresses include the '@' symbol. To send an e-mail:

(1) Open (log into) your e-mail account.
(2) Click on 'Create Mail'.
(3) Enter the recipient(s) e-mail address in the 'To' line on the screen. You can send the message to numerous people at the same time.
(4) If you would like to send a copy of the e-mail 'for information' to another person, add their e-mail address on the 'CC' line.
(5) Always give the e-mail a title by using the 'Re' box, e.g. Mrs G Granger F/F.
(6) When this information is in place, you are ready to start typing your message into the big blank box; you are often able to format the text so that you can send it in your preferred font, size or colour.
(7) When your message is complete, click on 'Send'.

If you wish to send the recipient a file already on your computer, you can send an attachment. Your ISP will provide instructions on how to attach files. In most cases you will need to click on the paperclip icon. Then a list of the documents on your computer will appear. Click on the file you want to send and it will be attached to the e-mail. Most e-mail accounts limit the size of the files that you can send as attachments. If you plan to send multiple documents, you may need to send them individually. E-mails with large attachments can take up to five minutes to send; those without attachments are normally sent in seconds. With some e-mail accounts you will receive confirmation that the e-mail has been sent; others only send notification if the e-mail was not successfully sent.

Instant messaging

Many of the free e-mail providers allow you to use instant messaging with other people with access to their services. This service is provided free of charge once their software is loaded on to your computer. When the account is set up, simply log on to the instant messaging program using the same login name and password as for your e-mail account.

When Instant Messaging is used in a dental practice, each part of the practice can be included in relevant communications. Each time you receive a new message your computer will make a sound to attract your attention. Alternatively you can set it to flash discreetly on the screen. As implied by the name of Instant Messaging, the message that you send arrives immediately. E-mails may take a few minutes to arrive, so urgent information should be sent as an instant message.

To add other people to your messaging account you need to know their e-mail address. You then simply add a contact to your account and an e-mail will be sent to them to confirm that they wish to be added to your list. When the person next signs into their messaging account, they can add you to their contacts by simply clicking to accept you as a contact.

Each time someone you have included as a contact signs into the instant messaging, you will be notified and able to send them an instant response message. The advantage of instant messaging over e-mailing is that you do not need to keep entering the e-mail address, or even click on reply. You can keep the message conversation open all day, or for as long as both people are signed in. Your conversation will be shown on the screen, so you will have a record of what has been sent.

Once you are confident about using these communication channels, they make a positive contribution to the smooth running of the practice, making it possible for information to be shared quickly and easily at all times.

Chapter 10
Dental Terminology

Dental charting

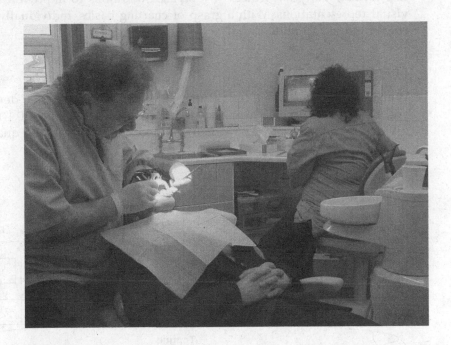

Dental charting is a technique developed by dental professionals to keep a permanent record of each patient's dental care by mapping:

- dental history;
- oral hygiene standards and home care instructions given;
- tooth abnormalities;
- x-ray findings;
- gum health;
- proposed treatment;
- future treatment plans.

When charting, the dentist and nurse work together, the dentist making a systematic clinical assessment of the patient's dental needs, which are spoken out loud for the nurse to record in the strange language that is regarded by many patients as one of the mysteries of dentistry. This chapter aims to provide new receptionists with the information they need to interpret dental charts.

The charting of existing conditions provides basic information for an accurate, comprehensive treatment plan. A dental chart notes the condition of all teeth present and teeth missing. It records the condition of all oral soft tissues, and the prescription for current treatment needs. Each assessment must follow the same sequence and requires clean, dry teeth, good lighting and x-rays.

Before computerisation all dentists used the international dental chart format shown in Figure 10.1. Although computerised systems are based upon this format, many have their own stylised additions to improve the chart's visual representations. With a grasp of charting basics, individually tailored charts are easy to understand.

Charting basics

When charting, the nurse uses letters, numbers and symbols to denote past and required treatments over each tooth. As shown in Figure 10.1 the chart divides the mouth into four quadrants and each tooth in the quadrant is

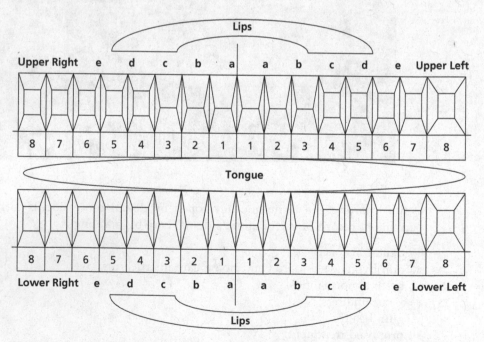

Figure 10.1 Standard paper chart.

allocated a space on the chart. It is important to note that the chart represents the mouth as the dentist views it, so for charting purposes the patient's right is charted as left. The chart illustrates the *five* surfaces of molars shown on the chart as 8, 7, 6 and premolars shown on the chart as 4 and 5.

The front teeth are shown with four surfaces; canines are represented on the chart as 3, and the incisors as 1 and 2. Deciduous teeth are represented with the letters a, b, c, d, e. During a new patient assessment, charting begins with general evaluation of the gums for presence of calculus on the teeth. Grading is from 1 to 3 where 3 is heavy calculus. Next the mouth is examined for missing teeth. A line is placed horizontally on the chart across any missing teeth. Enamel/dentine enamel/pulpal fractures are then observed and noted. A periodontal probe with millimetre gradations is inserted into the gum where it meets the tooth. The probe is gently pressed down to measure how far down each tooth's root the gum is secured to the tooth. The attachment depths referred to as 'pockets' are noted on the chart. The dentist then examines the soft tissues of the tongue and cheeks, before assessing the condition of each surface of each tooth present.

When examining the teeth, the dentist will call out the notation of the tooth by stating its position in the dental arch and will use the following terminology to describe its condition.

Sound: The tooth is dentally fit
Cavity: The tooth needs a filling
Filling: A filling is in place
Missing: Previously extracted
Crown: Previously crowned

When referring to fillings the dentist will name the surfaces of the tooth included as follows:

Occlusal = The biting surface of molar and premolars
Buccal   = The surface of upper or lower teeth nearest the cheek
Labial   = The surface of incisors and canines nearest to the lips
Lingual   = The surface of lower teeth nearest to the tongue
Palatal   = The surface of upper teeth nearest to the palate
Mesial   = The surface of all teeth facing towards the front midline
Distal   = The surface of all teeth facing away from the front midline

Charting shorthand

When there is a need to share information about particular teeth between dental professionals, teeth will be shown within their quadrant with the appropriate abbreviations. These abbreviations may differ slightly from dentist to dentist, depending on the dental software package they use and the dental school they graduated from. Some of the most commonly used

Table 10.1 Charting abbreviations.

Abbreviation	Meaning
AUG	Acute ulcerative gingivitis
BW	Bite wing = intraoral x-ray
DO	Distal occlusal
F/-	Full upper denture
-/F	Full lower denture
F/F	Full upper and lower dentures
FGC	Full gold crown
GI	Gold inlay
MO	Mesial occlusal
MOD	Mesial occlusal distal
OH	Oral hygiene
OPG	Dental panoramic tomograph = extraoral x-ray
P/-	Part upper denture
-/P	Part lower denture
P/P	Part upper and lower dentures
PJC	Porcelain jacket crown
PE	Partly erupted tooth
PPC	Porcelain post crown
RF	Root filling
S&P	Scale and polish
TBX	To be extracted
UE	Unerupted tooth
#	Indicates a fractured tooth or filling

abbreviations are listed in Table 10.1. These abbreviations are then shown in conjunction with the notation of the relevant tooth as follows:

$\underline{8}|$	TBX	Upper right 3rd molar to be extracted
$\underline{4}|$	#	Upper left 1st premolar fractured
$\overline{}6$	MOD	Lower left 1st molar requires a filling, incorporating its mesial, occlusal and distal surfaces
$1|$	PJC	Lower right 1st incisor requires a porcelain jacket crown

It is essential for receptionists to be able to read dental shorthand. A list of the practice's preferred abbreviations should therefore be included in the reception manual.

Glossary

Abrasion Dental abrasion is the term used when teeth have been physically worn away. A major cause of dental abrasion is poor brushing technique or brushing immediately after consuming acidic products, as acid-softened enamel is more susceptible to abrasion.

Accident In terms of health and safety legislation an accident is an unplanned, uncontrolled event with the potential to cause harm.

Aggressive behaviour Behaviour characterised by a physical or verbal attack. The aggression may be directed outwardly to others, or inwardly towards the self, in which case it can lead to self-destructive actions. Aggression can be the result of emotional conflict or frustration, or at times the means by which the aggressor exerts their will over others.

Assertive behaviour Behaviour in which you express your thoughts, opinions and needs without undermining the thoughts, opinions or needs of others.

At arm's length government bodies Created by the Department of Health, at arm's length government bodies' such as the Modernisation Agency, Special Health Authorities and Executive and Non-executive Agencies are responsible for the development of NHS services.

BDA Good Practice Scheme The Good Practice Scheme provides practical self-audit tools to enable practices to comply with current legal requirements and nationally recognised standards of good practice. Practices are required to meet 97 standards and to gather 52 pieces of evidence to demonstrate compliance with these standards.

Benchmark Benchmarks are specified standards used to measure current performance and identify any future improvements required.

Best practice The term 'best practice' refers to the identification of aspects of procedures that have produced outstanding results so that the best features of those procedures can be adapted for use in other situations.

Bridges Bridges are units of false teeth, fixed to natural teeth to fill a gap. A bridge may take the place of one or more missing teeth. The results can be functionally and aesthetically excellent. With careful maintenance a well-made bridge can last many years.

British Association of Dental Nurses The BADN is the UK's only recognised professional association for dental nurses in the UK.

British Association of Dental Therapists The BADT is the representative organisation for dental therapists in the UK.

British Dental Association The BDA is the professional association and trade union for dentists in the UK.

British Dental Hygienists' Association   The BDHA is the national professional association for dental hygienists in the UK.

British Dental Practice Managers Association   The BDPMA is the representative body for dental practice managers in the UK.

British Dental Receptionists' Association   The BDRA was formed to give receptionists in the UK a voice within the dental community.

Care coordinator   This role was developed to reinforce the work of clinicians when explaining complicated treatment options to enable patients to make informed choices about their oral care.

CEREC   CEREC (Sirona Dental Systems) is a system for making ceramic crowns, onlays or veneers in a single appointment in the dental chair.

Certificate in Dental Radiography   A qualification offered jointly by the Dental Nurses' Examining Board, the College of Radiography (COR) and the British Society of Dental and Maxillofacial Radiology (BSDMFR).

Charting   Dental shorthand used to record details of the condition of patient's oral tissues, in particular recording past, current and future treatment requirements.

Civil law   The law that applies to the rights of private individuals as opposed to the law that applies to criminal matters.

Clinical Audit   Formally introduced in 1993 into the NHS as an activity of Clinical Governance, clinical audit is a process seeking to improve the quality of patient care through systematic reviews of care provided against explicit criteria to enable clinicians to implement changes to enhance care standards.

Clinical dental technician   A dental care professional (DCP) registered with the GDC and permitted to make dentures for patients under the prescription of a dentist.

Clinical Governance   The term used in the NHS and the private health-care system to describe a systematic approach to maintaining and improving the quality of patient care.

Clinical Governance Kit   The BDA's Clinical Governance Kit is a practical guide for implementing essential quality assurance measures in dental practices.

Communication chain   The communication chain defines the communication process using the analogy of a chain, as the success of communications is dependent on a series of interlinked activities.

Confidentiality The ethical principle and legal right that a physician or other health professional will hold secret all information relating to a patient, unless the patient gives consent permitting disclosure.

Consent Consent is an implicit or explicit permission given by a person legally capable of consenting. Consent may be given by words or acts, or by silence when silence implies agreement. Consent to dental treatment must be the result of the patient being able to make an informed choice between treatment options.

Continuous professional development Dental professionals are required to commit to their continued professional development by meeting criteria for lifelong learning set by the GDC.

Criminal law Criminal law is the branch of law in which the state defines crimes and provides for their punishment.

Cross-infection control Cross-infection is the transmission of disease-causing germs from one patient to another, or from the patient to the dentist, or vice versa. This is prevented by Universal Precautions, so named because they are followed for all patients.

Crowns Crowns are caps made to fit over existing teeth. They are often recommended following root fillings to protect the teeth when their strength has been compromised by the extensive decay and infection that may have been present.

Curricular framework Within dentistry the GDC specifies a curricular framework setting out the knowledge and skills required by dental care professionals to hold GDC registration.

Customer care Measures taken to ensure dental patients experience high-quality non-clinical services to support clinical aspects of their care.

Data Protection Act This Act specifies legal requirements for the accuracy, storage and maintenance of information held about individuals.

Dental bodies corporate Dental bodies corporate are dental companies registered with the GDC and permitted to provide dental care to the public.

Dental care professional This term refers to ancillary members of the dental team qualified and registered with the GDC.

Dental Code of Practice Ethical standards set for dental care professionals and enforced by the GDC.

Dental Complaints Service The DCS was set up under the supervision of the GDC to respond to patients' complaints about dental treatments or dental care professionals.

Dental Industry Training Institute Under the supervision of the British Dental Trade Association, this organisation provides training for members of the dental trade.

Dental nurse The nurse's role is to assist dentists, therapists and hygienists in the provision of dental treatments, whilst maintaining the best possible level of patient comfort and safety during their visit.

Dental Practice Board: Special Health Authority The DPB is an 'at arm's length body' under the 2004 NHS structure.

Dental root planing When gum is inflamed, a pocket is formed between the tooth and gum. Root planing involves the use of scalers in the gum pockets to clean away the plaque that has built up there.

Dental technician Dental technicians are important members of the dental team who make a wide range of dental prosthetics including crowns, bridges, orthodontic appliances and dentures.

Dental Technicians Association The role of the Dental Technicians Association is to represent dental technicians. The DTA played a major role in helping to prepare for statutory registration.

Dental therapists Therapists carry out certain clinical procedures such as simple fillings, extractions and fitting crowns. They can also take impressions and dental x-rays, treat patients under sedation and administer injections.

Dentists Act The Act of Parliament defining dentistry in the UK.

Dentures Dentures are an effective method of replacing missing teeth, by providing the patient with a removable appliance. Dentures restore appearance, as well as the biting and chewing function, although the main disadvantages with dentures are they are sometimes difficult to tolerate, and are subject to slippage during speech and when eating.

Difficult patients Patients are considered difficult when their behaviour does not conform to acceptable social standards.

Discrimination To offer individuals treatment or consideration based on class or category rather than individual merit.

Disposable income   Money that individuals have available to spend after all financial commitments have been satisfied.

Distal   Refers to the surface of a tooth furthest away from the midline of the face.

Duty of care   Duty of care is set in health and safety law as the responsibility to take measures to ensure the well-being of others.

E-mail   Electronic mail sent via the internet.

Empathy   Empathy is the ability to see matters from another person's point of view and to recognise their needs.

Endodontics – root canal therapy   An endodontist is an expert in advanced restorative treatment of the root canal, a process that involves removing the damaged pulp at the centre of the tooth and replacing it with a synthetic material.

Environmental health officer   Environmental health officers are employed by local authorities to enforce environmental health measures.

Ergonomics   The applied science of workplace equipment design to maximize productivity by reducing operator fatigue and discomfort.

Erosion   The destruction of tooth tissue through frequent exposure to sweet and carbonated drinks.

Ethics   In philosophy, the study and evaluation of human conduct in the light of moral principles. Moral principles may be viewed either as the standard of conduct individuals have constructed for themselves, or as the body of obligations and duties society requires of its members.

EU Directive   EU Directives are instructions from the European Parliament to member states, requiring them to enact specific laws.

Evidence-based dentistry   The application of techniques designed from the results of research in practice.

External customers   In marketing terms, external customers are the purchasers of goods or services.

Extractions   In modern dentistry extractions are regarded as treatments of last resort. Dentists will only remove teeth beyond restoration or when the patient cannot meet the cost of restorative treatment.

Fillings   Damaged or worn teeth can be restored with fillings. There is a range of materials in common use for this purpose, including amalgam (silver), gold and composite resin materials. The new composite materials offer alternatives to traditional metal fillings and look like natural tooth tissue.

Fissure sealants   A plastic coating applied to the biting surface of molar and premolar teeth to prevent decay forming in the pits and fissures.

Freedom of Information Act   On 1 January 2005 the Freedom of Information Act became law, giving the public a right to access certain information about public services, including dental services.

General Dental Council   The General Dental Council regulates dental professionals in the UK.

General dental practitioner   There are around 27 000 dentists providing dental care in general dental practices in the UK.

Gestalt   A structure so integrated that its overall value is greater than the sum of its parts.

Gingivectomy   A gingivectomy is a periodontal procedure to surgically remove excess gum tissue.

HOT management   Hands-on transactional management is based on a clear understanding of the skills and abilities required for staff to achieve their work objectives.

Hygienist   A dental care professional, trained to scale and polish patients' teeth and deliver preventive care through oral health education.

Implantology – implants   Under certain circumstances it is possible for missing teeth to be restored with implantology. The procedure replaces the tooth's root with a strong titanium post, on to which crowns or bridges can be fitted.

Inlays and onlays   Inlays and onlays offer alternative methods of repairing damage to teeth involving more than half of the biting surface. Made of porcelain or gold, they are cast to the exact shape of the tooth and bonded to the damaged area of the tooth.

Instant messaging   Instant messaging is a popular and useful way of using computers for sharing non-standard information with colleagues.

Internal customers   In marketing terms, internal customers are the providers of goods and services.

Job description   An outline of the tasks an employer requires their employees to perform as part of their normal working routines.

Labial   The surface of the front teeth closest to the lips.

Legislation   Legislation is the term used to refer to laws made by Parliament and enforced through the legal system.

Manufacturers' representatives (reps)   Sales people sent out by manufacturers to potential customers to raise awareness of their companies' products.

Marketing   A core activity of practice management, requiring high levels of visionary, technical, diagnostic and problem-solving management skills. The aim of marketing is to make your business the logical place for your customers to satisfy their dental needs, not just once, but over and over again.

Marketing mix   The marketing mix is a technique used to define the goods and services your customers want, so that you can develop the right product, at the right price, in the right place, for the right people.

Medical emergencies   Medical emergencies occur when a patient's general health gives rise for concern during a dental visit. Fainting and asthma attacks are the most common medical emergencies and can be easily managed when the dental team is first response trained. More serious medical emergencies may require the intervention of paramedics.

Medical history   Dental professionals have a duty to provide the most appropriate care for their patients. This requires knowledge of the patient's current and past general health, along with up-to-date information on any medication the patient is taking. Clinicians have a responsibility to ensure medical histories are verified and updated at every dental visit.

Mesial   This term refers to the surface of all teeth facing towards the midline of the patient's face.

Motivation   This term is used to describe certain types of behaviour. It can be described as a mind-set that influences our willingness to take action.

National Health Service   The NHS was instigated by Aneurin Bevan to provide health-care services free at the point of delivery, financed by central government and based on need.

Negative stroke   A negative interaction between people designed to communicate the message, 'I'm OK, and you're not OK'.

Negotiation   Negotiating is a form of communication designed to share facts, ideas, attitudes or opinions with the aim of changing the other person's point of view.

Non-assertive   Non-assertive describes behaviour in which an individual fails to stand up for their rights.

Occlusal   This term refers to the biting surface of a molar or premolar tooth.

Occupational health   Covers a vast range of subjects related to the well-being of people at work.

Operations manual   The practice handbook bringing together working protocols and practice policies.

Options for Change, O4C   Options for Change is a Government report published in 2003, recommending radical changes in the NHS.

Oral assessment   A full mouth assessment will establish what past treatments have been completed and current treatment needs. Unless there is any reason not to, a full set of radiographs are taken to complete an oral assessment. This process will generally take around 30 minutes.

Oral health promotion   Covers a wide range of activities carried out by every member of the dental team aiming to enable patients to understand how they can achieve and maintain a good level of oral health.

Oral surgery   Oral surgery provides treatments for a wide range of problems that can occur within the mouth. Most are related to the teeth, though some problems may involve the jaw or the gums.

Orthodontics   This specialist dental care concentrates on the alignment of teeth in the jaws to improve function and make home care easier for the patient. Orthodontists have a detailed understanding of how the teeth, jaws and face grow, and are skilled in the design, use and placing of braces and corrective appliances to correct the position of the teeth and jaws. In addition to improving a patient's appearance, they can also improve the bite (occlusion) of teeth. When teeth don't meet correctly, this is called 'malocclusion' and the orthodontist will correct this.

Ozone   Ozone is a form of oxygen, a natural biocide that effectively kills bacteria. Applied to the tooth surface it kills the bacteria that cause tooth decay, and sterilises the site so that, when the debris is removed, a filling material can be used to replace damaged tooth material.

Palatal This term refers to the surface of the upper teeth nearest to the patient's palate.

Periodontics – gum therapy Periodontal disease (also known as gum disease or pyorrhoea) is a bacterial infection in the gums and bone supporting the teeth. If not treated, this ongoing infection can destroy the bone around teeth, resulting in tooth loss.

Permitted duties The duties each member of the dental team is permitted to perform under the terms of the Dentists Act.

Policies Policies are pre-agreed plans made by management to influence and determine future decisions and actions.

Positive stroke A positive interaction between people designed to communicate, 'I'm OK. You're OK'.

Practice information leaflets (PILs) Since the early 1990s practice information leaflets or brochures have been used to communicate information about practice services and terms of business to patients. More recently paper leaflets are being replaced by practice websites.

Practice manager Practice managers are responsible for the day-to-day smooth running of the practice. Their duties include overseeing the observation of legislation relevant to dental businesses, such as employment law, health and safety, and data protection law, thus enabling the dentist to concentrate on clinical dentistry.

Practice rules Agreed procedures and protocols to promote teamwork. Usually set down in the practice handbook.

Primary care The first tier of health care provision, where patients refer themselves for care provided by dentists, doctors (GPs), pharmacists and opticians.

Primary Care Trusts (PCTs) There are 303 PCTs throughout England and Wales, each responsible for managing primary health services in their specific local area. They are responsible for ensuring that the services available meet local needs.

Proactive To act proactively is to plan and prepare in advance, to deal with future events, rather than responding after the event.

Procedures Procedures are series of steps taken to accomplish tasks. Consistency in patient care is achieved when standardised procedures are agreed within teams.

Prosthetics   Prosthetics are artificial body parts such as dentures.

Protocols   Protocols are the codes of conduct agreed with a team for inter-acting in specified circumstances.

Quality charter   A set of guiding principles for the standards of care a practice aspires to provide for their patients.

Quality cycle   The process of defining standards, measuring results and adapting working methods to achieve and exceed pre-set standards.

Quality management   Taking action to set aims, objectives and standards for services, then monitoring performance to standard.

Reactive   Acting in response to events.

Recall   Some practices send recalls to patients to let them know it is time for their routine dental assessment, whereas others rely on patients remembering to book an appointment when they are due.

Registration   Dentists and dental care professionals are required to register annually with the General Dental Council before they are permitted to perform acts of dentistry.

Retail representatives (reps)   Sales people from dental retail companies, through whom practices can purchase the products of a wide range of dental manufacturers.

Risk   In health and safety terms risk is a calculation of the likelihood of harm.

Robens Committee   The Robens Committee was set up in 1972 to consider how health and safety legislation could be made more effective. Their recommendations gave rise to the Health and Safety at Work Act 1974.

Root canal therapy   Root canal therapy (see Endodontics) is designed to correct disorders of the dental pulp – the soft tissue around the tooth that contains nerves, blood vessels and connective tissue. Teeth with abscessed, or infected, nerves were once removed with corrective therapy. Now, in 95% of these cases of pulpal infection, the natural tooth can be saved through modern endodontics procedures.

Royal College of Surgeons   The Royal College of Surgeons of England is an independent professional body committed to promoting and advancing the highest standards of surgical care for patients. It is situated at Lincoln's Inn Fields in London.

Safety   In health and safety terms safety is an absence of risk.

Scale and polish   After a dentist has made an assessment of the patient's treatment needs, if necessary, a scale and polish appointment may be made with the hygienist who performs thorough cleaning of the teeth and gums and provides advice on how to carry out effective home care procedures such as regular flossing and careful brushing.

Secondary care   Secondary care includes general medical services in hospitals and other locations. Services are provided to patients referred by primary care practitioners.

Self-regulation   The dental profession has the privilege of self-regulation under the guidance of the General Dental Council.

Six Key Principles for Ethical Practice   Guiding principles set down by the General Dental Council for dental professionals and dentists' conduct.

Six-pack   The 'six-pack' is the name given to the half-dozen most widely quoted health and safety regulations issued by the European Commission and introduced in Britain through six European Directives.

SMART objectives   SMART objectives are a technique for planning and measuring performance. Clear measurements of the success of any project are difficult to achieve unless the expected results are defined from the onset.

Specialist dentists   After qualifying as a Bachelor of Dental Surgery (BDS), or gaining an equivalent recognised qualification, some dentists choose to continue training and become expert in a particular procedure to offer specialist dental services to patients referred by other dentists.

Strategic Health Authorities   There are 28 Strategic Health Authorities, who provide links between the Department of Health and the NHS Trusts and Primary Care Trusts (PCTs). Their role is to support and monitor the work of PCTs.

Sterilisation   Sterilisation is the elimination of all bacteria, prions and viruses from a surface or piece of equipment. This is different from disinfection, where only organisms that can cause disease are removed by a disinfectant.

Terms of business   Terms of Business are a declaration of the terms under which the practice provides dental care to patients.

Tertiary care   Tertiary care services are highly specialised, and include intensive care units and neuro- and thoracic surgery. Highly sophisticated technology and facilities are required.

Tooth whitening Tooth whitening is a popular cosmetic procedure. A bright, white smile can make you look good and feel great. Patients who have experienced a tooth whitening transformation say that the procedure helps them smile with confidence.

Transactional analysis During the 1950s psychologist Eric Berne studied people's interactions and formed his theories of transactional analysis, which are to this day widely used to predict and explain human relationships.

Treatment plans and estimates Dento-legal requirements specify that patients must be given full and detailed explanations of treatment plans and estimates of costs.

Turnaround time The time it takes for a dental laboratory to complete a task and return the work to the practice ready for the next surgery stage.

Universal Infection Control Measures taken to prevent the transfer of disease-causing pathogens from one person to another by regarding each patient as 'high risk'.

Veneers Veneers are made of porcelain or plastic and are placed over the front teeth to change their colour or shape.

Vocational training A training scheme for new graduate dentists to enable them to further develop their skills under the guidance of an experienced mentor.

Waste Materials that dental practices need to dispose of. Waste is categorised as contaminated or special waste according to the risk it presents to individuals and the environment.

Wellness management Wellness management is a measurement of an employee's ability to work as assessed by an occupational therapist.

X-ray: radiographs Dental x-rays provide a picture of what is happening in areas not visible to the naked eye. Early signs of decay, impacted teeth, abscesses and bone loss from gum disease can all be detected on an x-ray.

Section 3
Planning and Managing Dental Services

Chapter 11
Managing People

The tactical management process

Managers working in modern, high-pressure business environments need a clear vision of where their practice is going and why. A clearly defined purpose is essential to success and provides managers with guidance, clarity and direction. When managers fail to recognise the purpose of their role, they become reactive and spend much of their time responding to situations rather than being proactive and making the best use of the resources available for the success of the business.

Large multinational organisations need complex management structures. Here the senior managers are directors, who are far removed from the company's day-to-day operations. They are strategic managers; their role is to decide what the company does and to identify ways to capitalise on opportunities that present themselves. With a clearly defined company strategy in place, it is then the role of tactical managers to decide how to use resources to achieve the strategic objectives.

Strategic managers	define WHAT the company's objectives are
Tactical managers	define HOW to achieve the company's objectives

Although dental practices are not multinational companies, it is essential that they have a management structure incorporating strategic and tactical management skills to prevent them from spending time firefighting rather than on fire prevention. In this way a two-level model of practice management is created: with the strategic management input from the practice owner(s) at the director level, and the day-to-day tactical management input of the practice manager. These roles are set out in Figure 11.1.

Practice management teams consist of directors and managers, all of whom need to work together to agree practice policies and procedures that the manager will implement in a fair and consistent manner. Managers and the directors must establish robust communication channels to ensure that information

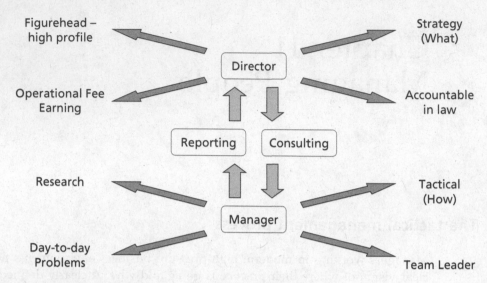

Figure 11.1 Management model for dental practices.

is shared on a routine basis, through reporting and consulting processes. In this way they support each other's roles and authority.

Many of today's practice managers were appointed in recognition of their seniority and loyalty to the practice; although they are highly experienced and skilled dental professionals, they may well have little or no formal management training or qualifications and benefit greatly when introduced to the tactical management process.

> The tactical management process is a staged approach incorporating essential management skills, enabling managers to adopt a structured approach to management. The approach requires managers to research, design, plan, implement, audit and evaluate their own and others' working activities. In this way a consistent and logical approach to management builds skills, defines best practice and facilitates learning from experience. The tactical management process requires the application of specific management techniques as shown in Table 11.1.

Skills and activities at each stage of the tactical management process

Initiation

This is a trigger setting a course of events into motion. Proactive management initiatives are triggered when managers consider the best use of resources to achieve the company's strategic objectives. Inevitably some triggers will require a reactive response, for example when new legislation is introduced and the manager needs to design compliance measures. Initiation is the point at which tactical managers recognise the need to take action.

Table 11.1 Tactical management process.

Stages	Actions and activities
Initiation	This is the point at which you recognise the need to take action.
Research	Before acting, the manager needs to systematically gather information to clarify objectives and how to achieve them.
Design	At this stage, the manager identifies results, in SMART terms that can be audited and evaluated at the end of the project: **S**pecific **M**easurable **A**chievable **R**elevant **T**ime measured
Planning	Here practical decisions of how to use resources to achieve the end result are made.
Implementation	At this point, the plan is put into action.
Audit	When the time measured period has elapsed, the objective information (hard facts and figures) specified in the SMART objectives are audited to assess the results.
Evaluation	Here subjective information (aspects of satisfaction and well-being) are considered.

Research

This is a systematic investigation of the facts, conducted before taking action to ensure that you don't blunder in blindly. At this point the manager assesses the resources available and begins to visualise the end result. As advocated by Steven Covey in his book *The Seven Habits of Highly Effective People*, they should 'begin with the end in mind'. Through a process of questioning and consideration of the information gathered, the manager increases their understanding of what is required and how to achieve the strategic objective.

Design

Here the project's framework (WHAT needs to be done) is identified. At the design stage the manager creates the strategy, preparing the way for the tactical planning stage when the practicalities of HOW to proceed are made. The design needs to be detailed and specific: the saying 'To be terrific you must be specific' highlights the importance of SMART objectives at the design stage that can be audited and evaluated at the appropriate time. Take a dental practice where the principal dentist needs specialist-nursing support; Table 11.2 shows how you would use the model described. With SMART objectives in place it is possible to create a detailed action plan.

Table 11.2 SMART objectives.

SMART	Actions	Project considerations
Specific	Set objectives	To recruit a part-time, qualified, implant-experienced dental nurse.
Measurable	State how much, when, who	To recruit the nurse for 12 hours per week, commencing in 4 weeks' time, and to work for £9.00 per hour.
Achievable	Consider if the specific and measurable aspects are realistic and assess the chances of achieving them	How likely is it that we can recruit a qualified nurse with experience of implantology, to work for 12 hours per week at £9.00 per hour? How likely is it that such a person could start work in 4 weeks' time? This may lead to adjustments to the specific and measurable aspects.
Relevant	Identify how the above contribute to the achievement of the specific objectives	At this point you are re-checking effectiveness of the design.
Time measured	Time the project; define when results will be audited and evaluated	Here you must specify when to measure your results by assessing the objective and subjective impact of the initiative's results: ■ objective results: an audit of facts and figures; ■ subjective results: an evaluation of the satisfaction and well-being of those involved.

Planning

Planning is the act of formulating a programme for a definite course of action. At this stage the manager makes decisions on how to achieve the end result and allocates resources. Here practicalities are agreed, for example how to attract applicants for the position, who will conduct the interviews and determine their criteria and format. Here the initiative progresses from being a concept to reality.

Implementation

Implementation is the process of putting the plan into action. It is important to keep a record of events for analysis, noting all aspects where expectations were either exceeded or unattained. Recording this for later analysis will enable the definition of best practice for future activities.

Audit

This is a review and examination of objective information (facts and figures) to test the adequacy and effectiveness of progress towards specific objectives. This will take place when the time measured aspect of the SMART objectives has elapsed, when the manager refers back to the objectives specified at the design stage.

Evaluation

In this context the evaluation is essentially a set of philosophies and techniques to determine if a programme 'works'. It is a field that has emerged using the audited information to assess the value of the final results, compared with the results identified at the design stage of the process.

The tactical management process is a structured, logical and methodical management technique enabling managers to take a considered approach towards management initiatives. The technique uses a staged approach, breaking down the activities at each stage into sections that lead into each other and leaving an audit trail for final assessment of the success and value of management projects.

Motivation

The word 'motivation' is often used to describe certain sorts of behaviour. A nurse who works hard and with enthusiasm may be described as being 'highly motivated'; whereas a less enthusiastic team member may say she is 'finding it hard to get motivated'. Such statements suggest that motivation has a major influence on our behaviour.

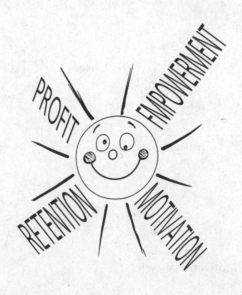

Motivation can be defined as a mind-set that influences our willingness to take action. While it is easy to see what people do, it is much harder to guess at *why* they are doing it. For example, our hard-working nurse may be working hard because she wants to earn a bonus, or it could be that she really enjoys her job. She may be striving to impress her manager or just want to do a good job.

Theories of motivation

Many studies have attempted to predict the extent to which we can be motivated to take certain actions. Psychologist Abraham Maslow argues that motivation is driven by an internal drive to satisfy a hierarchy of needs; this is termed an inside-out theory as it argues that our behaviour is influenced by the extent to which our internal needs have been met. Another key theory, suggested by Frederick Hertzberg in the *Harvard Business Review* in 1963, predicates on the premise that motivation is the result of the workplace environment and culture. This is an outside-in theory. In practice, managers recognise the importance of meeting the team's internal and external needs to sustain a good level of motivation.

Since it is part of a manager's job to get their work done through others, managers need to understand what motivates each team member so that they can direct them to work towards the goals of the practice following the motivational cycle shown in Figure 11.2.

Motivation is the result of an interaction between the needs, incentives and perceptions of individuals. When the correct balance is found between these factors, the result is positive motivation. The balance, however, is individual to each person and so a subjective process requires managers to use a wide range of interpersonal skills. Since motivation is a very fragile commodity yet

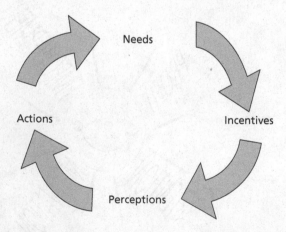

Figure 11.2 Motivational cycle.

essential for the achievement of practice goals, numerous studies have led to the creation of guidelines to enable managers to create and maintain a well motivated team.

Expectancy theory

> Here motivation is attributed to incentives tailored to the needs of the individual. This theory is based on four premises:
>
> (1) People have preferences for various outcomes or incentives available to them.
>   *(People know what they want.)*
> (2) People hold expectations about the likelihood that action on their part will lead to an intended outcome.
>   *(People know what to do to get what they want.)*
> (3) People understand that certain behaviours will be followed by desirable outcomes.
>   *(People understand the consequences of all behaviours they could adopt.)*
> (4) The action a person chooses will be determined by their expectations and preferences at that time.
>   *(This is not fixed and will respond to individuals' circumstances.)*

Work motivation has considerable importance in the workplace. It concerns the direction, intensity and persistence of work behaviour. There are a number of theories as to what can be done to enhance motivation. Some psychologists view motivation as a product of innate human need, others as a calculation based on 'How can I get the most out of this situation?'.

When managers recognise how individual team members are motivated, they are able to design win–win incentive schemes to achieve the practice goals whilst satisfying the needs of individual team members, as shown in the following example.

'There have been many changes in dentistry over the past few years, and the expansion at my practice has meant increasing the team and introducing new, often challenging, work procedures. We have always endeavoured to create the right working environment, where people can apply their theoretical and practical understanding to produce outcomes that have commercial, social and personal value. The team are given opportunities to acquire new knowledge and skills to enhance career and personal development. In doing this, individuals are rewarded for enhancing their knowledge value and the collective knowledge of the practice, and for contributing to the practice's core values.'

It is possible to introduce something akin to a 'Green Shield Economy' in which staff members are recognised and rewarded for their contributions to the practice. The team are very receptive to the concept of 'reward bundles', because these give them choice and flexibility as individuals as opposed to a blanket system of reward for the whole practice. Some staff could opt for an extra two days' holiday for the year rather than a pay increase if family commitments meant that additional annual leave was more beneficial than a pay increase. In showing this adaptability and co-operation as employers, you strengthen the relationship with team members.

Flow theory

Winner of the Thinker of the Year Award 2000, Mihaly Csikszentmihalyi, a professor and former chairman of the Department of Psychology at the University of Chicago, has devoted his life's work to the study of what makes people truly happy, satisfied and fulfilled. Csikszentmihalyi (pronounced 'chick-sent-me-high-ee') is chiefly renowned as the architect of the notion of flow in creativity; people enter a flow state when they are fully absorbed in activity during which they lose their sense of time and have feelings of great satisfaction. Csikszentmihalyi describes flow as, 'being completely involved in an activity for its own sake. The ego falls away; time flies, every thought and movement follows inevitably from the previous one, like playing jazz. Your whole being is involved, and you're using your skills to the utmost'.

When working in a busy, well organised and efficient dental practice, it is easy to achieve the flow as described by Csikszentmihalyi. The days and weeks simply fly by and team members feel they are achieving something worthwhile. On the other hand, when team members are not fully occupied at work, motivation nosedives, leading to conflicts between team members.

The eight rules of motivation

To build a robust and motivated team environment, managers must make sustained efforts to lead by example within a disciplined atmosphere of respect and based upon these rules of motivation.

(1) *Be motivated yourself*. Enthusiasm is contagious. When managers have a positive, 'can do', attitude and show they are giving 100% to their work, they set a positive tone to work culture, which team members will buy into.
(2) *Select people who are highly motivated*. When a new member is introduced to the team, the dynamics shift. Research carried out by psychologist Tuckman identified four stages through which groups work before they become a team. When recruiting into the team, great care should be taken to ensure the new recruit shares your practice values and is temperamentally suited to work as part of your team.
(3) *Treat each person as an individual*. When people are treated with fairness and consistency, they feel positive and motivated to contribute to the team. Clever management is responsive enough to maintain

fairness and consistency, whilst recognising people's individual needs and responding to them. Policies based on openness and honesty can maintain fairness alongside responsiveness.

(4) *Set realistic and challenging goals.* The satisfaction realised through achieving challenging goals can be a major source of pride and motivation. In contrast, the sense of failure resulting from an inability to achieve unrealistic goals will cast a shadow over the team and undermine individuals' desire to work wholeheartedly towards future goals. Managers should have a realistic idea of what each team member is capable of, and work with them to expand their skills.

(5) *Remember that progress motivates.* Make sure your team receives regular feedback on their progress towards stated goals. Making good progress and not knowing about it can be as demotivating as failing to make progress towards practice goals.

(6) *Create a motivational environment.* If creation of a motivated environment depends upon meeting people's needs, the manager needs to organise the practice to avoid unnecessary obstacles to the achievement of tasks. Every part of the team should be encouraged to work together and to recognise and enjoy each other's successes.

(7) *Provide fair rewards.* Although money is not the only reward dental professionals have need of, if their earnings do not cover their bills, they will have to find better-paid work. In this respect dental employers need to compete with employers from other sectors. Even so, high pay and motivation do not always go hand in hand. A fair salary plus other rewards for loyalty and achievement should be provided in line with pre-set criteria to ensure they are distributed fairly and meet the team's expectations. Such rewards could be pension plans, private health insurance, and trips out. If a bonus system is to be used, great care must be taken to ensure it is based on clearly measurable criteria to avoid demotivating conflicts.

(8) *Give recognition.* In a busy practice it is easy to find you are not taking the time to speak to some members of the team when a problem has arisen. Managers should make a point of noting the quality of every team member's contribution and, at least once a week, taking time out to show they are aware of the standard of their work, rather than waiting for the annual appraisals to discuss performance.

In the workplace, no theory stands alone to explain team motivation. The common denominator in all of these theories are two drivers:

Needs: the need to be free from hunger and extremes of temperature, and to be safe and pain free.

Benefits: the desire to achieve more, e.g. wealth, respect, happiness, love, friendship.

Everyone is driven by a combination of these drivers, which influence our action and priorities.

Leadership

Leadership is the process by which people influence the behaviour of others. When listing the most influential people of the day, trend-setting celebrities who regularly send ripples across society will be high on the list, with political and religious leaders often less influential than charismatic figures such as Bob Geldof and Jamie Oliver. If leadership is best measured by results, some of the most influential people are not obvious leaders but those who apply attributes such as beliefs, values, ethics, character, knowledge and skills.

Although holding the position of manager gives you the authority to accomplish certain objectives in the practice, this authority does not make you a leader . . . it simply makes you the *boss*. Leadership differs in that it makes the followers *want* to achieve objectives, rather than simply bossing them around. For the smooth running of the practice, managers need to apply a proactive balance of management and leadership qualities.

For people to give their best, they need to understand their contribution to the practice. When managers regard their teams as allies in the achievement of practice objectives, they treat them as individuals and nurture them to realise their potential within the team. Nurturing people is like planting a garden: to produce a good crop, gardeners start with healthy plants; to provide the best possible start, they need to know the conditions each variety of plant needs and to tend them carefully. If you use this approach with people, the possibilities are endless.

Synchronised leadership

Synchronised leadership focuses on the 'Power of Four'. The four elements are shown in Figure 11.3. Alone, each of these elements has positive effects on groups, but together they create a *gestalt*, in which their combined effects are greater than the sum of the individual parts.

Vision

The practice's mission statement sets out a clear vision of the purpose and nature of the practice, which is used to define the practice's standards and

VISION	CHALLENGE OF SKILL DEVELOPMENT
The practice has a clear destination and pathway to reach that destination	CPD with measurable results
A SENSE OF BELONGING	FUN
To know where you fit into the overall picture	

Figure 11.3 The Power of Four.

attitudes. For example, this could state, 'We are an ethical private dental practice with up-to-date equipment and well-trained, happy staff, providing high quality dental care with an emphasis on prevention. Our aim is to provide quality dental care in a modern, well equipped practice, delivered in a caring and relaxed environment.' With this type of clarity, managers can make day-to-day operational decisions and work with the whole practice team to set service standards and procedures consistent with realising the vision.

Skill development

Through an ongoing learning programme for all the team, the practice provides continuously improving patient services and increased team confidence, enabling the team to view themselves with pride as dental professionals.

Managers need to take the lead in skills development by conducting learning needs according to how best to achieve the practice's mission and with consideration of the learning styles within the team. The educationalists Honey and Mumford produced a manual of learning styles in which they identified the learning environments that best suit different types of learners, whom they categorised as activists, reflectors, theorists and pragmatists.

- **Activists** thrive on the challenge of new experiences and like to be fully involved. They revel in coping with crises, but once the excitement has died down they look for new challenges because they get bored with routine work. They enjoy working with others, but like to be the centre of attention.

  Activists learn best from having new experiences, problems and opportunities to tackle. They like to be thrown in at the deep end, with tasks they think are difficult and can use their own ideas for problem solving. They will gain less from learning experiences requiring them to work on their own a lot, e.g. reading or writing lots of notes, when they have to take a back seat and not get involved or need to follow instructions to the letter with little scope for manoeuvre.
- **Reflectors** like to collect all the facts and look at situations from all angles. They are cautious and dislike reaching a definitive conclusion until they have thought it through thoroughly. Reflectors prefer to take a back seat, observing and listening to other people before they make their own move. Reflectors learn best when they can do things in their own time, without having to meet tight deadlines. They need time to think before acting and to review what has happened and think about what they have learned. They are not suited to learning opportunities in which they are pressured or rushed from one activity into another. They do not like to be in the limelight, i.e. taking a leadership role, or being the centre of attention.
- **Theorists** approach situations and problems logically, working step by step to integrate their observations into complex theories. They tend to be perfectionists and like to fit all the facts neatly into their rational scheme of things. They favour theories, models and systems, and reject anything

that doesn't fit their rationale. They like to be certain of things and feel uncomfortable with intuitive judgements.

Theorists are happiest in learning situations where the structure and purpose are clear and they know what is required of them, when they have time to think ideas through logically, can see logical patterns and are intellectually stretched. They learn less when pushed into doing things without knowing the context or purpose and feel intellectually out of tune with the others, especially activists.

■ **Pragmatists** like to get straight to the point and act quickly and confidently on ideas that attract them. Pragmatists are essentially down-to-earth people who like making practical decisions and solving problems. They are more comfortable with things that they know are going to work. Pragmatists learn best when working on tasks with obvious practical advantages and when they can quickly see the results of their efforts. They like to try things out for themselves, with feedback from a creditable expert. They learn less when they are not able to see any point in their tasks, do not receive a 'pay-off' for work completed or do not have clear instructions, or have no chance to practise new tasks.

A skilled manager offers adequate learning opportunities compatible with team members' learning styles; can keep people motivated; and boosts team morale while lowering stress levels, raising productivity and increasing the team's problem-solving skills.

A sense of belonging
Measures to make each member of the team feel involved and integral to the team's success create a sense of belonging. This is emphasised during the team meeting where all members of the team are actively encouraged to participate by sharing their views and opinions. A sense of belonging features as the third level of Maslow's hierarchy of needs. Maslow argues that people need satisfaction of progressive needs within a five-levelled hierarchy, beginning with their physiological needs. Having met the latter, they progress to fulfil their need for safety and security, and then on to the need to belong within a social structure. With this need satisfied they are able to progress on to fulfil their need for self-esteem and accomplishment. When managers identify where each team member is in the hierarchy, they are able to provide the means to progress them to the next level.

A sense of belonging is dependent upon people knowing how they fit into the overall design of the practice, having a clear role, and being confident that they have the skills and knowledge to fulfil that role.

Fun
Enjoying yourself is as important during work as during your leisure time. All work and no play is not the formula for a successful working environment. To increase staff morale and team spirit an element of fun is required.

This could take the form of taking the team out for lunch as a reward every so often, or a day out for the sole purpose of strengthening the team relationship. Great people motivators have fun with their teams. They have fun working hard and playing hard, because they understand the healing power of laughter and the motivational power of having fun whilst working hard.

Leadership and productivity

What is the link between leadership and productivity? Katz and Khan have carried out a number of studies in leadership and have found that there are three dimensions of leadership consistently related to productivity.

(1) *Assumption of the leadership role*. Managers who took a clear leadership role were found to get better results than those who assimilated themselves into the group.
(2) *Closeness of supervision*. High-producing supervisors provided staff with training and guidelines, then gave them the freedom to do their jobs in their own way.
(3) *Employee orientation*. High-producing supervisors were consistently found to be more employee- and less production-focused. They provided a clear and supportive management structure, identified the competences of employees and gave considerable freedom to the competent workers.

This study found the democratic leadership style to be the most productive, in which leaders discussed projects with the team, set aims, objectives, borders and boundaries, provided training in the necessary skills, and then left the team to work as they saw fit.

What workers need from their leaders

Studies have found over 75 key components of employee satisfaction. Having trust and confidence in leadership has been identified as the single most reliable predictor of employee satisfaction, and effective communication by leaders in three critical areas shown to be the key to winning employee trust and confidence:

- helping employees understand the practice's objectives;
- helping employees understand how they contribute to achieving the practice's objectives;
- sharing information with employees on progress towards the practice's objectives.

So, in a nutshell, you must be *trusted* and you have to be able to *communicate a vision* of where the practice needs to go.

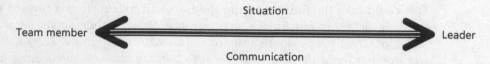

Figure 11.4 The four major factors in leadership.

Four factors of leadership

There are four key factors of leadership as shown in Figure 11.4.

Team members

Leaders must be flexible enough to be able to adapt their style to respond to the leadership needs of each team member. For example, a new employee requires more supervision than an experienced employee. A person who lacks motivation requires a different approach from one with a high degree of motivation. You must know your people! The fundamental starting point is having a good understanding of human nature, such as needs, emotions and motivation.

Leader

Leaders need an honest understanding of who they are, what they know, and what they can do. Leadership requires two-way trust and confidence. To be successful you have to convince your followers, not yourself or your superiors, that you are worthy of being followed.

Communication

Two-way communication is the essence of leadership. Much of it is non-verbal. For instance, when you 'set the example', you communicate to your team that you would not ask them to do anything you would not be willing to do yourself. What and how you communicate either builds or undermines the relationship between you and your team.

Situation

What you do in one situation will not always work in another. You must use your judgement to decide the best course of action and the leadership style needed for each situation. For example, you may need to confront an employee about their inappropriate behaviour, but if the confrontation is too late or too early, too harsh or too weak, then the results may prove ineffective.

Leaders are not born. Leadership is an achievement gained through consistent hard work and dedication. The methods that managers use to lead their team can either greatly strengthen the team spirit or completely destroy it. An effective leader must have the benefit of the whole team supporting them, as many initiatives that the practice will embark upon require a whole team effort to succeed. This not only increases staff awareness of the procedures in place but also strengthens the levels of communication demonstrated and builds upon the existing team structure. The responsibilities of the leader will change from time to time and therefore the necessary skills and attributes will also alter. For the leader to remain effective they must actively demonstrate awareness of personal competence. This encourages self-assessment, which will highlight any weak areas and allow for improvements to be made.

Postscript

'No institution can possibly survive if it needs geniuses or supermen to manage it. It must be organised in such a way as to be able to get along under a leadership composed of average human beings.'

Peter Drucker, 1993

Staff selection

In the vast majority of cases, when practices have staff problems, those problems could have been avoided by the application of advanced staff selection skills. With hindsight, managers often say they missed clues in the application or interview processes which should have alerted them to the potential for future problems. Selecting new staff should always be a careful process, as applicants may well put enough spin in their application to make it misleading, hiding information about tell-tale employment gaps, periods of extended sick leave and job hopping due to an inability to build healthy workplace relationships. It is well known that people exaggerate at job interviews. However, the scale of exaggeration and the resulting problems are an increasing cause of concern.

Unlike large companies with whole departments of personnel management experts, dental practice managers have fewer opportunities to hone their staff selection skills. This means it is important to make the most of every opportunity to learn from your recruitment experiences, building necessary skills by developing written selection processes and procedures, then recording and evaluating end results for policy development purposes.

Creating structured recruitment processes begins with careful consideration of the aims and objectives at each of the following stages, so that appropriate actions can be defined.

Identify your staffing requirements

The staff selection should be guided by policy, procedures and intuition. This begins with the production of an organisational chart, giving a visual display of the practice structure and where each team member fits in. From this you can build your job descriptions and person specifications. When interviewers have a clear definition of the person they are looking for, they can recognise them when they appear for interview. With this in place, recruitment becomes a matching process in which the manager looks for the following attributes to find the best fit for the position being filled.

> *Hard attributes*:   relating to the applicant's knowledge, skills and experience
>
> *Soft attributes*:   relating to the applicant's personality and temperament

The advertisement

The tone and presentation of your advert will determine the number and quality of applications. It is advisable to invest in a larger, upbeat advert giving details of the position, the practice website address, and a closing date for applications. Your advert should instruct applicants on how to apply for the position.

The choice of publication will be dependent upon the position being advertised. Local papers are the most logical choice for recruiting nurses and receptionists, whereas hygienists and dentists are often recruited through adverts in their professional associations' journals or the dental press. Other recruitment routes are internet sites, which are growing rapidly in number and can be found using a search engine, or dental recruitment agencies.

The application

For short-listing purposes, an application form is the best application method as it should gather the same information about each applicant. A CV can be used to support applications if necessary. It is vital to ensure that your selection procedures have due regard for equal opportunities requirements. This means each applicant must be offered the same chances to show how he or she meets your pre-set criteria for the position. (These should have been clarified to applicants in the application pack sent in response to their initial enquiry.) In response to application enquiries you should send out a standard response including:

> *The job description*. This should cover:
>
> - general information about the practice;
> - the main purpose of the job;
> - working locations and conditions;
> - reporting procedures;
> - salary;
> - benefits.

The person specification is an outline of the ideal person for the job, setting out the physical, psychological and experiential factors that interviewers will be looking for. This will cover:

Skills:	training, aptitudes, qualifications, experience and knowledge
Sociability:	interpersonal skills, reliability, leadership skills
Personality:	intelligence, judgement, maturity, interests
Physical:	agility, stamina, special sensory requirements

Each of the above should be classified as essential or desirable, and questions to assess applicants' suitability in each area should be included on the application form and used as part of the short-listing process.

Make sure you send each applicant the application form with guidance for its completion, giving applicants an idea of how much detail is required in their responses. You should give the closing date for applications and the date on which interviews will take place.

Your practice brochure will give applicants a feel for the practice and should detail information about your location and on parking availability and public transport services.

Always give at least one week's notice of the interview appointment. When scheduling interviews allow equal and ample time. Allow for delays and time for the panel to discuss applications directly after the interview.

Short-listing

Short-list the applications by matching applicants to attributes for the position. Having awarded scores for the attributes required, set qualifying scores for interviews. Write to the successful applicants with an interview appointment and details of how the interview will be conducted.

Interview

You cannot expect to change the person you employ. You can train them, but you cannot fundamentally change their personality. Look for outward signs of their character observable in their appearance; for instance are they clean, tidy and well groomed? Grading of these aspects of the applicant's appearance should be recorded on the interview record.

The interview can be supplemented by references from tutors and previous employers. There is no obligation on a previous employer to provide a reference, and indeed references offered by applicants may not be genuine or accurate. It is a good idea to check with the author by phone to validate any document you have been presented with. You may learn a lot.

The interview is your opportunity to ask about relevant documents such as work permits or education and professional certificates. Whenever possible, ask to see originals, which, with the permission of the applicant, you can copy and retain for checking.

It is vital that employers check information provided by applicants. The simplest way of checking a person's background is by asking probing questions at the interview. This should include their hobbies and interests to make sure information they have provided is accurate.

Interview questions

There is a wide range of interviewing methods to choose from. Your method of choice will be influenced by the person specification you are trying to match. Irrespective of the method chosen, the interviewers must:

- Ask relevant questions.
- Ensure that all questions relate to selection criteria.
- Keep the interviews consistent.
- Give applicants details of terms and conditions of employment.
- Tell applicants when they can expect to hear about the results of the interview.

Keeping applicants in the picture is an indication of your professionalism.

Before the interview you should prepare an interview pro forma, to be followed for each person interviewed. This could include the following questions:

(1) Why are you applying to us?
(2) Ask for examples of:

- how they work;
- organisational skills;
- coping with different demands and tasks;
- working under pressure;
- working with difficult people.

(3) Ask for medical information and if it's OK to request a medical reference.
(4) Ask about availability for work.
(5) Ask how much they know about the practice, then proceed to fill in the gaps.
(6) Ask if they have any questions for you.
(7) Finally ask, '*If* you were to be offered the job, would you accept?'

The interview room

Interviews are nerve-racking experiences. Try to avoid setting the room out in a confrontational style such as sitting facing each other over a table. Instead ensure that the room layout is relaxed and friendly. Open with preliminary chat to establish rapport, and then ask if you can take notes, which should be kept brief during the interview and expanded upon directly after the applicant has left the room. Show that you are giving your full attention to the applicant when they are speaking directly to you. During the interview, the balance of proactive communication should be 80% applicant, 20% interviewer.

Collect references

Dental employers must ask applicants to provide criminal records clearance. Three levels of certificate are available from the Criminal Records Bureau, depending on the nature of the work being applied for. In certain cases, the certificate will provide details of spent and unspent convictions. Always ask applicants for permission to approach referees; it is essential to follow through, sending standard reference forms (with a stamped addressed envelope) to the personal and professional referees named in the application.

The job offer

When you have made your selection decisions, successful and unsuccessful applicants must be informed. The provisional job offer you send is the basis of an employment contract so always state if the offer is subject to medical information and references.

The job offer should provide details of:

- the starting date and time (as discussed during the interview);
- salary;
- place of work;
- hours;
- pay arrangements;
- induction procedures.

Include a letter of acceptance for them to sign and return to you.

An effective selection process will have been designed to provide the information required in order to enable managers to assess the applicant's suitability for the position advertised and to establish whether the applicant is capable of doing the job to the required standard, whether they are well motivated and how they will fit into the existing team.

New staff inductions

Dental practices, like any other business, can find that their staff are their greatest asset or are a major obstacle to achieving the highest standards of professionalism. To ensure staff are an asset, great care should be taken in selection and in integrating them into the team. To enable staff to realise their full potential, managers need to implement a staff development programme to provide guidance and support. This programme should define the practice's objectives, set standards for conduct and skills development and introduce personal development plans.

Personal development plans are at the heart of staff development. Members of all professions are required by their lead bodies to keep their skills and knowledge up to date through a programme of continuous professional development (CPD). CPD is a personal commitment to improve your capabilities throughout your working life; it is about knowing where you are today and where you want to be in the future, and planning how to get there.

A structured staff development programme begins with a staged induction process, leading into the first appraisal interview during which a development plan is agreed along with measures for assessing progress.

The induction process

The aims of the induction process are to enable new team members to adapt to the culture of their new workplace and set a tone of cooperation and motivation for working relationships. The induction begins with the letter of appointment, which should say the time you want them to arrive on their first day, where they should go and the name of the person to ask for on arrival.

The next step is to prepare for their arrival by making sure the receptionist is expecting them and knows what instructions to give them on arrival. It is a good idea to prepare their working space if possible, make a locker available for their personal belongings, and have a day-1 induction pack ready and waiting for them.

Timetable an hour or so to spend with the new recruit at the beginning of their first day so that you can put them at their ease; maybe ask them to arrive as late as 10 am so you can deal with any urgent tasks before they arrive. During this first meeting make sure that they know to whom questions should be addressed and that they understand the basic principles of:

- hours of work;
- sickness notification and certification requirements;
- welfare arrangements: kitchen, coats, first aid, fire instructions, lunch hours and cover;
- holiday booking procedures and principles;
- punctuality;
- discipline;
- conduct;
- standards of dress;
- personal phone calls;
- cooperation and flexibility;
- quality and quantity of work;
- general housekeeping;
- safety requirements.

To develop their understanding of their new post, outline their role and its overall importance to the practice, then introduce them to immediate colleagues and outline their induction programme. Experience shows that little of what staff are told on their first day is remembered, especially if they are ill at ease on their first day in a new job. Therefore the manager should deal first with matters affecting their health and safety. Provide other information on a 'little and often' basis to build confidence and understanding gradually. When possible, support verbal information with written documents that they can keep. Make sure they have a copy of the practice organisation chart (making certain they are included on this).

Induction timetable
The induction timetable should be as follows.

Stage 1
On the first day of their employment provide an induction pack containing:

- the job description;
- the practice's mission statement;
- the practice's service commitment;
- details of the induction training programme;
- the practice organisation chart;
- the health and safety policy;
- fire instructions;
- important telephone numbers;
- practice information leaflet.

In addition:

- make introductions to colleagues;
- familiarise them with fire regulations, and with staff welfare arrangements such as toilets and kitchen;
- invite questions on any subject to do with their employment;
- start on-the-job training.

Stage 2
At the end of week 1, arrange to hold an interview to discuss their training and experiences during the first week. At this time you can introduce the practice manual containing the practice's policies. This interview also gives you the chance to evaluate your induction procedures and make any changes deemed necessary for future recruits.

Stage 3
At the end of week 4, arrange a further meeting to review progress. This review process is essential to build confidence, trust and efficiency, and confirms your interest in their progress. A further review should then be planned for the end of the probationary period.

Induction checklist

When complete, the induction process will ensure new staff are fully aware of practice policy for:

■ hours of work;
■ holiday booking procedure and principles;
■ sickness notification and certification requirements;
■ welfare arrangements such as toilets, kitchen, coat racks, first aid, fire instructions;
■ lunch hours and cover;
■ smoking breaks;
■ punctuality;
■ discipline, conduct and standards of dress;
■ personal phone calls, inbound and outbound;
■ cooperation and flexibility;
■ quality and quantity of work;
■ housekeeping and safety requirements;
■ their role and how it contributes to the overall picture;
■ training programme and review steps.

The induction is one of the most important training phases for new staff, and although it is time consuming it is a worthwhile investment in team development.

Staff appraisals

The term 'appraisal' is becoming increasingly unpopular because it is considered too formal for small dental practices. The term 'personal development review' (PDR) is regarded as more congenial. PDRs are opportunities for employees to sit down with their managers and explore ways in which the individual and the practice can work together to achieve the highest possible standards of excellence. Staff can discuss with their manager their work achievements, support learning and development needs.

The objective of the appraisal is to link the practice's objectives with the skills and achievements of the team. It is an ongoing process, to set objectives for the coming year which will be appraised at the year's end. Through this process, managers will identify learning and development needs, agree a personal development plan and evaluate the effectiveness of previous learning and development initiatives.

Conducting an appraisal

Where, when and who is involved in the practice appraisals systems will be outlined in practice policy. A suggested appraisals system is as follows:

■ Set the time and place for the interview and enclose an appraisal form.
■ The employee is asked to score their performance on the appraisal form and give this to the appraiser before the interview.

- The initial interview should take between 30 minutes and 1 hour.
- The appraiser should make bulleted notes of the discussion during the interview and action any points agreed with targets and time scales.
- Following the interview the appraiser should complete the feedback section of the appraisal form and forward to the employee for their signature to confirm their agreement. Two copies of this should be made, one to be given to the employee and one to be kept in their personnel records.

Skills for appraisers

For the appraisal process to realise its full potential, appraisers need a range of communication and coaching skills. They need to understand the importance of allowing employees to voice their opinions, even if they do not like what is said. This is best achieved by asking open questions to set the scene and focus attention on the employee. The manager needs to keep the employee focused on relevant issues, addressing one issue at a time.

Giving and receiving criticism during appraisals

At times, appraisers will need to give and receive criticism. The appraisals must not be used as part of the disciplinary process. Employees subject to disciplinary measures should not be appraised until disciplinary matters are settled, nor should any disciplinary measures be instigated through the appraisal. Never introduce criticism not already addressed through the management system. If there is a need to revisit problem areas, do not make this the first item for discussion. Make sure the criticism is valid and recognises any improvements since the last discussion of the problem.

Focus on the behaviour rather than the individual. If you have a staff member who is clearly unhappy or going through a difficult time, the appraisal should be postponed and the underlying problems addressed. Never postpone issues unnecessarily. If there is praise to be given, say it or take appropriate steps now, and keep appraisals an open process that you share with your staff.

Troubleshooting

If, for any reason, there is a failure to reach agreement in the appraisal, a second short interview should be set within two or three days to revisit the area of disagreement. If this interview fails to provide a solution, a third party should be introduced as an arbiter and their decision is final.

Arbiter
It is advisable to name one person to be arbiter for a range of appraisals and another to be called upon if the first arbiter is directly related to the initial failure to agree.

Development plan

The desired outcome of staff development measures is the creation of a culture of whole team professionalism, with each member of the team committed to their continuous professional development. Dental teams are made up of people from widely different academic backgrounds, so it is essential that development opportunities are drawn from a wide range of learning activities. Some of these will be specific to particular team members whereas others will bring the whole team together for learning.

Although each person's development plans will be specific to them, activities should fall within agreed measures to ensure equality of opportunity within the team. Equality is achieved through a practice policy for team development. This policy should provide a framework of relevant activities to be personalised during the appraisal interview, creating each person's professional development plan for the coming year.

Staff development takes place on a formal and informal basis. We all continuously learn from everyday work experiences. At times we find we lack specific skills or knowledge. Development plans aim to anticipate the skills and knowledge needed for the future, so plans can be made for development activities. Thinking about the future and identifying potential needs enable you to choose to participate in the formal and informal learning opportunities shown in Table 11.3.

Having identified the range of learning opportunities available, the practice manager needs to set benchmarks for staff development and define a plan for each member of the team, clarifying their participation in the following activities:

- development of a professional CPD portfolio;
- appraisals;
- inductions;
- staff meetings;
- ongoing in-house staff training in specific areas;
- attendance at training courses (minimum one per year);
- attendance at specified short meetings when no courses are available;
- membership of professional associations;
- on-site one-day health and safety, first aid and other necessary courses;
- peer review.

Table 11.3 Learning opportunities.

Formal learning opportunities	Informal learning opportunities
Courses and training events	Reading (books and journals)
Qualifications	Staff meeting
Staff inductions and appraisals	Belonging to groups and associations
Mentoring	Trade videos
Projects	Networking

The rewards for 'getting it right' with staff development are many. When people feel able to perform well and know that their input to the team is valued and appreciated, an upward spiral of achievement and work satisfaction is established bringing immeasurable benefits for the dental team, the practice and most importantly the patients.

Chapter 12
Planning and Managing Dental Services

Policy development

Consistent management requires a clear vision of where the practice is going. In today's business environment, managers need to secure an appropriate balance between profitability and compliance with legal and ethical obligations. When agreed ways of working in the form of practice policies and procedures are in place, practices are more likely to run smoothly and equitably. Some policies, such as those concerned with health and safety, are legal requirements. For other areas of the practice, policies should be written to ensure that everyone is working in unison.

Policies should not be written by managers and handed out to the team: the whole team should be involved in policy development. When involved from the start, people have a better understanding of what they should be doing and why. Practice policies should be living, working documents, not simply produced and filed away. Once in place, the practice manager ensures policies are observed. Once agreed, a copy of each policy should be distributed to each team member to read, sign and keep.

> Every practice should have written policies on Clinical Governance, cross-infection control and emergency procedures, to name but a few. The purpose of policies is to clarify team roles and responsibilities.

Policies should reflect the practice's values and philosophy, providing benchmarks and working instructions. Beginning with a statement of purpose, each policy provides a framework for decision-making and working procedures for its area of activity. With policy decisions in place, a consistent and equitable approach can be adopted when there are conflicts of interest which could potentially result in conflicts within the team. Policies should be flexible enough to allow discretion in their implementation, provided that the basis of that discretion is built into the policy.

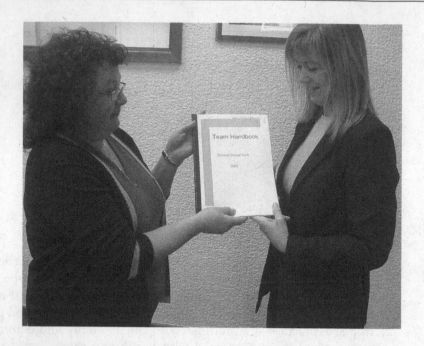

Policy writing

To make the practice vision reality, the manager needs to agree policies to move the practice forwards. Policy making is strategic management built on the following series of decisions about the areas covered by the policy outlined in Table 12.1:

- the *purpose* of the policy;
- the *scope* of the policy;
- the *working instructions* for the observation of the policy;
- the *review* process.

The working instructions section of the policy should be posted in the area where the work is carried out. For instance the procedure for calling the emergency services should be placed next to every phone in the practice. Working instructions provide useful guidance to people required to perform tasks that are not normally part of their working routines, and ensure they work safely and to standard. When a new team member joins the practice, these working instructions provide excellent backup for on-the-job training and ensure that procedures are carried out by new staff in the same way as by established staff.

Discussing policies and procedures at practice meetings gives everyone a chance to have their say and to feel that their views are incorporated into practice routines. Policies are kept up to date and relevant when discussed regularly at practice meetings. Clear and agreed policies empower managers to

Table 12.1 Outline policy.

Area	Coverage
Purpose	This is an outline of your strategic aims. For example, the purpose of this policy is to ensure that this practice provides and maintains a safe and healthy working environment, equipment and working procedures.
Scope	Here a statement of who will be involved in the observation of the policy. For example, the practice principal has overall responsibility for health and safety in the practice. Every team member has a duty of care to behave in ways that secure their own health and safety and that of others affected by their work activities. All accidents and spillages should be reported to the practice manager at soon as possible.
Working instructions	List the actions required to achieve the aims of the policy. For example, with regard to protective clothing: all protective equipment provided for staff and patients must be used as instructed. Heavy duty gloves to be worn when cleaning sharp instruments and when using hazardous chemicals.
Review	Identify the review process. For example, this policy will be reviewed annually by the practice managers and immediately if circumstances change. Any changes or updates will be discussed in a practice meeting.
Agreement	The policies should be signed and dated by the employer and employees.

take decisive action should the behaviour of an employee be in contravention of an agreed policy. The manager can bring the situation to the notice of the employee and require them to act in line with policy in future. If it came to a point where disciplinary action was required, the manager could refer to the policy and use it to check that the employee had understood and was able to perform as required. In this way, a remedial action plan can be clearly defined.

Communicating policies can be used for team building. For example, practising emergency and first aid procedures as a team can remind everyone how important and fulfilling it is to work together and communicate. There are many ways to communicate practice policy to the team and ensure everyone is working towards the same goals and is fully aware of what is required of them and others. Talking through procedures builds team spirit and teaches colleagues to respect and listen to each other's point of view. These measures will produce written policies and procedures which should be subjected to

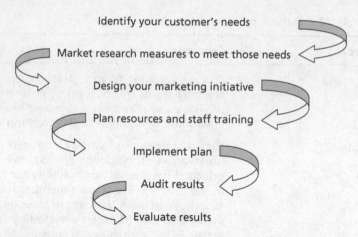

Identify your customer's needs

Market research measures to meet those needs

Design your marketing initiative

Plan resources and staff training

Implement plan

Audit results

Evaluate results

Figure 12.1 The marketing process.

regular reviews and updates, providing the framework for consistent good practice.

Marketing dental services

Many busy practices believe they do not need to carry out any marketing because they have more than enough patients. However, marketing is not simply about attracting new patients: it is about ensuring that you develop a profitable business by meeting the needs of your external customers (patients who purchase dental services from you) and your internal customers (team members who provide the services you sell to patients).

Marketing covers every activity of management. Many activities of marketing are included in your Clinical Governance requirements. In Figure 12.1 you will see how the tactical management process covered in Chapter 11 applies to the management of marketing initiatives.

The marketing mix

Marketing requires visionary, technical, diagnostic and problem-solving skills. Through the application of the marketing mix (also known as the 5Ps) managers can make their practice the logical place for customers to fulfil their dental needs, not just once, but over and over again. The marketing mix is a technique used to define the goods and services your customers want, so you can develop and **promote** the right **product**, at the right **price**, in the right **place**, for the right **people**. When you know what your customers want, you can design and coordinate the right services.

Marketing skills

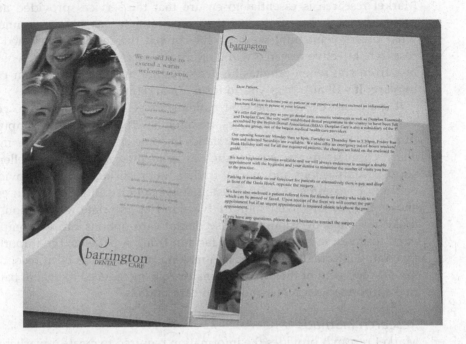

Successful marketing begins with a marketing plan, in which your marketing objectives are set out in SMART terms. The vision originates from the practice business plan in which aims and objectives are stated, to be shared with the whole team. The energy and motivation needed to drive marketing initiatives forward can arise from visualising the results, as described by golfer Jack Nicklaus.

'I never hit the shot even in practice, without having a very sharp, in-focus picture of it in my head. It's like a colour movie. First, I see the ball where I want it to finish, nice and white and sitting up on the bright green grass. Then the scene quickly changes and I see the ball going there, and its path, its trajectory shape, even its behaviour on landing. Then there is a sort of fadeout and the next scene shows me making the kind of swing that will turn my images into reality'.

Many marketing initiatives fail to reach their potential due to a lack of clarification or planning. Other initiatives are rejected at the planning stage, due to lack of time, skills or resources. The truth is, if you do not have the time to plan an initiative, it is unlikely you will have the time to see it through. Until you have a clear vision and a specific plan, you just have a vague idea which cannot be managed or measured. A standard technique used to create clarity is the development of SMART objectives. In this way details are clarified and indicators set for measuring progress towards achieving them.

Market research

Market research is essential to ensure that the services provided are what patients want to buy and what the team wants to provide. We cannot know what others want until we have interpreted the results of targeted market research. Effective research will identify your customers, and show why they buy from you when purchasing decisions are made and who your competitors are. It will also help you to form a marketing plan.

It is a mistake to assume your patients are getting the most from your services since consumer behaviours are often habitual. Customers simply repeat purchases they know and understand. In some cases your patients may purchase cosmetic dental goods, such as whitening and tooth jewellery from shops, beauty salons and market traders, not realising that you provide them or do not recommend them. Customer behaviour can be changed; evidence shows that, when given sound advice and appropriate information, people make reasoned decisions. Because dental care options can be complex, we need to invest in putting the full facts in front of patients; the importance of providing information for decision-making processes has been recognised by the development of the care coordinator role, introduced to enable patients to make informed decisions about oral care options.

Research methods

Market research provides the information required to create a marketing plan to balance the needs of the internal and external customers.

> There are numerous market research methods widely used in dental practices to gather information relevant to the development of dental services such as:
>
> | | |
> |---|---|
> | Questionnaires: | used to establish customers' opinions and perceived needs |
> | Postal surveys: | sent out with recalls, returned at patients' appointments |
> | Observation: | watching and listening to customers on the practice premises |
> | Happy sheets: | ask 'How well are we doing?', on a scale of 1–5 |
> | Suggestion boxes: | in the waiting room or front hall can be valuable |
> | Census information: | the demographics of your area |
> | Focus groups: | asking targeted groups for feedback and ideas |
> | Monitoring competitors: | to understand what others do and to find ways to compete |

Listening to patients

If the only feedback from patients is complaints, then a more holistic patient feedback programme should be introduced such as the '3Cs' system, through which patients' compliments, comments and complaints are gathered.

Comments

There are many ways of gathering patients' comments, each of which have a role in understanding their points of view. It's always a good idea to invite informal verbal feedback from patients, provided there are also opportunities for them to give unfavourable feedback without putting themselves on the spot. Anonymous feedback sheets (happy sheets) will gather useful information, provided they are distributed to everyone, not only to patients you expect to give a glowing reply.

Even comments about the practice colour schemes or the books in the waiting room provide important insights into how patients view the practice. If we listen carefully to our patients, they will tell us what we need to know to continually improve our services.

Complaints

Complaints handled well can improve the relationship between the customer and provider. When the customer's concerns are addressed promptly and effectively, formal complaints can be avoided. On rare occasions the relationship between a patient and the practice will break down and the patient will go elsewhere. However, most situations can be resolved by taking appropriate action as soon as the problem becomes evident.

NHS in-house complaints procedures were introduced for dental practices during April 1996, following the recommendations of the Wilson Report. Practices were required to develop effective in-house complaints procedures, following a defined code of practice. During 2005 this programme was developed further to include procedures for responding to complaints from non-NHS patients.

Details of the complaints handling procedures are included in the patient's complaints section in Chapter 5.

Compliments

When patients are delighted with our services and products, we need to take careful note of exactly what exceeded their expectations. When we know what we are doing right, we can do more of it.

Sometimes when a patient is delighted by our services, it is because an individual member of staff has 'gone the extra mile' for them. The service culture in the dental team is important and should be built into our procedures, rather than being based on an element of chance. Service standards, which are set and enforced, ensure consistency in patient care.

Preparing the team

Successful businesses create a balance between the needs of the internal and external customer groups. Even with a clear vision, marketing plans will fail to reach their potential if, for any reason, the team are not able to make appropriate contributions to success. Managers need to assure each person has:

- the necessary equipment;
- the necessary skills;
- the right motivation.

The necessary equipment

Having the right tools for the job can make light work, whereas working without the tools or with faulty or outdated equipment will invariably impact on the quality of work performed.

The necessary skills

Before asking anyone to perform new tasks, make sure they have the appropriate training, support and feedback mechanisms to build confidence and enthusiasm. It is essential to include training provisions in any marketing plan. Details must be provided of how tasks will be performed and working instructions written in order to make first-generation information available so as to eliminate the 'Chinese whispers effect' that occurs when work instructions are passed on verbally.

The right motivation

Motivation is a key factor in marketing success and each team member responds differently to the motivators you might build into the plan. You need to understand this and ensure that each person will be able to gain something of value from participating in the initiative, be it increased patient satisfaction or pay incentives.

Although there is undoubtedly truth in the old saying, 'If you want a job done, give it to a busy person' there are nevertheless limits to how much work one person can do. If your team were fully stretched for all of their working time, it would be naive to add to their workload and expect them to achieve on an additional initiative with enthusiasm, consistency and accuracy. When each team member is fully involved in a marketing initiative and can see the results of their work, marketing initiatives can bring teams to life. People have a pragmatic approach to work tasks and need feedback on their efforts. Thus, by involving them in all aspects of the initiative they become more likely to 'go the extra mile' to achieve success.

Analysis of research information

When analysis of information gathered from research initiatives includes the factors shown in Figure 12.2, insight into the needs and expectations of internal and external customers is gathered. With this insight and the involvement of the team, you are ready to form your marketing plan. As a group, discuss the research findings, reach agreement on interpretations and brainstorm ways to use the results. Besides adding depth to your marketing, you will ensure that team needs are brought into the open for discussion and the whole team can buy into initiatives.

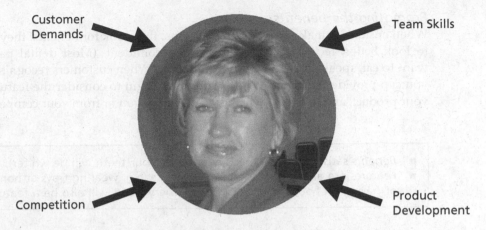

Figure 12.2 Information that needs to be gathered in order to form a marketing plan.

> **The marketing plan**
> Colonel John 'Hannibal' Smith of the 'A Team' was famous for saying: 'I love it when a plan comes together'. All managers can identify with this sentiment. When a well constructed and implemented plan produces the desired results, the rewards are most satisfying. Marketing plans begin with a strategy: an outline of *what* you want to achieve. With this in place, the technical details of *how* you will achieve your goals can be added.

In the retail sector, billions of pounds are spent every year on the presentation of goods and services; window dressing is a key aspect of selling. In the same way the promotion and presentation of dental goods and services must be aesthetically pleasing and fire the imagination and enthusiasm of purchasers.

> When designing promotional campaigns for professional services, you have to decide whether you need to educate or inform customers. It is important to be clear about this.
>
> - *Education* is appropriate when goods and services are new to the customer and they need to learn about the potential benefits.
> - *Information* is appropriate when customers are already familiar with the product and you want to show them why they should buy it from you.

Promoting the benefits

When customers make purchasing decisions, they look for benefits: they want to look better, feel better or become more confident. (Most dental patients want to eat, speak and smile with confidence.) When customers recognise that you can provide the benefits they want, they begin to consider the features of your product, and to decide whether to buy from you or from your competitors.

- *Benefits* satisfy the customer's needs (e.g. your teeth will be whiter);
- *Features* are about how the product works (e.g. wearing trays at home or having a I hour treatment in the surgery). Cost will also be a feature.

The marketing campaign

Marketing campaigns begin with the identification of your target customer groups so that you can design a marketing campaign to appeal to them. Then you need to decide how to put your information in front of them at a time when you can respond to their questions. Wherever possible, use visual images. They have an effect comparable to talking to someone in a particular tone of voice. The visual tone of printed materials and signs creates impressions of the product or service. Just as you may well judge a book by its cover, patients judge the practice on visual impressions based on the appearance of the practice.

When considering image you should look at the following from the patient's point of view:

Practice name:	Does it match the image you want to portray?
Practice appearance:	Does the practice appeal to the type of patients you want as customers? Is the building well maintained, comfortable, clean and tidy? Is the decor coordinated and consistent?
Information for patients:	Do you have up-to-date patient information leaflets? How are they distributed? Are all your services shown? Can patients discuss their dental needs and aspirations with a member of the team?

The customer focus

The tactical management process should be used to develop customer-focused services. This will involve staff training to ensure that all activities are consistent with the service standards promised to your customers.

For your patients (the external market) this may include the need for staff to:

- smile when interacting with patients;
- establish initial eye contact, even when too busy to speak to the patient immediately on their arrival;
- whenever possible call the patient by name;
- give individual attention when dealing with patients;
- keep patients informed and reassured;
- use body language to show interest;
- show respect, both to patients and colleagues;
- be well groomed, clean and tidy.

For your team (internal customer market) this will be a fair working environment in terms of:

- equitable salary levels;
- clear contracts and job descriptions;
- induction procedures and appraisals;
- staff being kept informed;
- recognition of their achievements.

Job satisfaction is the direct result of others showing acceptance, appreciation or pleasure in what you are doing.

Setting aims and objectives

The aims and objectives are an integral part of any marketing plan. So too are the methodology and criteria with which you measure your success in achieving them. At the time identified in the time measured aspect of your SMART objectives, you will need to gather information to assess results. This information will be qualitative and quantitative.

Qualitative information

To assess your initiative you highlight experiences during the initiative to say what went well, what you will do differently in future and how the results you have achieved have affected teamwork, morale and patient comfort in your practice.

Qualitative information is subjective and looks at how customers:

- think and feel about the initiative's results;
- experience your goods and services;
- make decisions to buy.

This type of information is gathered by asking open questions such as:

'How helpful did you find our reception team?'
'What did they do that made your visit more comfortable?'

Quantitative information

When the initiative is completed, an audit should be completed to analyse results in the format of reports, tables and graphs to compare the investment made with the results achieved.

> Quantitative information is objective and looks at measurable facts such as:
>
> ■ statistics, budgets and sales;
> ■ how many other practices in your area offer the same service;
> ■ which appointments are the ones that are most frequently not kept.

Pricing your product

To state the obvious, businesses must sell their goods and services for more than it costs to produce them. Not to do so is financial suicide (in the same way that charging more than customers can pay will lead to financial ruin). To manage income and expenditure appropriately requires managers to:

■ make the most economical use of resources;
■ have in-depth knowledge of the market, the competition and the needs of purchasers and providers.

Pricing is likely to be the toughest decision you need to make and it is important that you follow a structured process, as shown in Figure 12.3, to ensure that you give value to the customer and make a profit for the business.

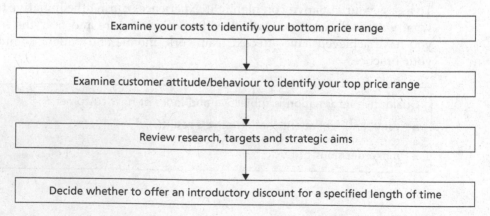

Figure 12.3 Pricing process.

Making a profit

When setting your price you need to look at other suppliers to ensure that you are competitive. However, you must be sure you are comparing like with like, as price is not the only factor customers consider in the decision-making process. They are also looking for guarantees, safety and quality. If your price is higher because you are adding one of these commodities, make sure you are highlighting this in your promotional materials.

Budgets

The very nature of business is investing to accumulate. When it comes to marketing, you can do very little without an investment (budget) to support your initiative. The manager's role is to ensure that a good return is secured on business investment. At the planning stage, the manager needs to produce projections of the expected return: best and worst case scenarios within the measurable aspect of the SMART objectives. Market research establishes how you can get the maximum spending power from your budget, and maximum benefits from the investment.

Marketing is about people; it is about attracting people, getting them to buy, and making sure they are happy enough with their purchase to come back for more. Marketing consists of many different activities: sales, advertising, customer service, the product, pricing and discounts, reputation, strategies and much more. Which of these elements is the key to success? Which should you emphasise and how can you coordinate these elements into a successful marketing initiative? As with any aspects of management, the key to success is in balancing the needs of the customers and the business through having a deep understanding of your customers' needs and thinking innovatively to meet those needs.

Risk management

The Management of Health and Safety at Work Regulations 1999 (MHSWR) provide a framework for managing health and safety, supplementing the more general duties in the Health and Safety at Work Act 1974. The former require employers to undertake the management tasks associated with risk control: risk assessment, planning, organising, controlling, monitoring and reviewing control measures; cooperation and coordination with other employers; involving employees; ensuring employees' health and safety training; and getting competent help.

The MHSWR require employers to conduct regular risk assessments to identify hazards and resulting risks to employees and other people affected by their work activities. The Act defines hazards as the potential for harm, and risks as the likelihood and severity of harm. Like the Health and Safety at Work Act 1974, the MHSWR require employers to assess risks, but the MHSWR are much more specific and require employers to:

- assess risks to employees;
- assess risks to others who may be affected by work activities;
- clearly identify the measures needed to protect individuals;
- review the assessment and make changes as necessary.

To conduct a risk assessment, the employer needs to investigate and identify what could go wrong and identify preventative measures. When practices employ more than five people, the employer must keep written records of assessment findings, identifying anyone considered to be at risk.

A team approach to risk assessment is most effective, with practice managers responsible for implementing required measures by setting policies and procedures supported with appropriate training for all team members.

The aim of risk assessments is to recognise and control the risk of injury or violence in the workplace arising from the work environment.

Dental employers should carry out and record risk assessments for all work activities. Such assessments will cover:

Autoclaves	Fire	Slips, trips and falls
Children	First aid	Smoking
CoSHH	Ionising regulations	Staff training
Cross-infection control	Lone workers	Stress
Display screen regulations	Noise	Vaccinations
Electricity	Nursing and pregnant mothers	Violence to staff
Emergency drugs and equipment	Personal protective equipment	Waste
Ergonomics	Sharps	Water
		Young people

The responsibility for identifying the possibilities of harm is shared between employers and employees. The Health and Safety at Work Act provides a legal context of shared responsibility. Even so, some practices only take action to protect their staff in reaction to incidents. It is not difficult for practices to assess risks and put preventative measures in place to protect staff.

When conducting risk assessments you must:

- Look for hazards.
- Decide who might be harmed.
- Evaluate the risks and decide if existing precautions are sufficient.

Look for hazards

Look for hazards that could result in harm, such as the layout of the practice, office equipment, how reception staff contact colleagues in other parts of the building in case of emergency, and how and when moneys are banked. By reviewing past incidents, assessing staff attitudes to safety measures, and discussing ways staff might be 'at risk', remedial action can be identified.

Decide who might be harmed

Once hazards have been identified, consider who is at risk. Once the risks have been identified, those at risk usually welcome positive measures for their protection. It may be senior managers who need convincing of the value of developing safer working procedures. Commitment from the top is essential and this should take the form of a policy statement supported by action.

Evaluate the risks

To evaluate risks, in order to determine whether you need to act to reduce the risk, consider how likely it is that each hazard will cause harm and how severe the harm could be. Even with measures in place, some risks remain. For each significant hazard you need to decide whether the risk is high, medium or low. Where the potential and likelihood for harm are assessed as high, measures must be taken immediately to either cease the activity or bring the level of risk down to one that is acceptable.

Record your findings

If you have fewer than five employees, you are not legally required to keep written records of risk assessments but it is advisable. However, employers with five or more employees must record the findings of risk assessments.

Employers are also required to inform employees of findings and show they have:

- made proper checks;
- established who is at risk;
- dealt with all obvious and significant hazards;
- taken reasonable precautions;
- reduced risks;
- kept detailed and careful records. Health and safety inspectors can request to see your risk assessments and details of precautionary measures taken.

Allocate responsibility

The employer is ultimately responsible under health and safety law. However, it is advisable for the employer to appoint a workplace health and safety coordinator to ensure that the policy is enforced and safety measures are implemented. Incidents and accidents should be reported to this person, who will be responsible for debriefing and making appropriate reports and recommendations.

Review your assessments and revise as necessary

Strategies for managing risks at work should be monitored and incidents recorded. At times this will require a sensitive approach towards employees who have been injured or otherwise harmed as the result of a workplace incident. Full details of the events leading up to the incident and the employee's part in it need to be established and recorded, even though people involved may be experiencing feelings of loss or reduced self-esteem. Without this information, any revision of safety measures may be ineffective.

Introducing changes

Risk reduction measures should include training for members of the team considered 'at risk'. Training should include revised safety guidelines and practice policy. It is important to provide employees with adequate preparation and support when their working routines have been amended for safety reasons. Once measures to control workplace risks have been agreed to ensure that high-risk activities are controlled, staff must be trained to manage any remaining risks.

The aims of the staff training are to:

- Make staff aware of potential risks and preventative measures.
- Enable staff to identify threatening situations in their earliest stages.
- Clarify safe reactions in threatening situations.
- Familiarise staff with safe working procedures.

The aims of training will be to ensure that the whole team are able to take appropriate and reasoned steps to ensure their own safety and the safety of others in the workplace.

As in all forms of management, health and safety management must be structured and tangible to be effective. In small organisations such as dental practices, the pressures of running the practice can result in health and safety considerations being overlooked. Health and safety law requires employers to determine safety strategies tailored to their own workplace. Adherence to measures outlined in the MHSWR enables practices to achieve good standards of health and safety, which are beneficial for everyone involved in practice activities.

Financial management

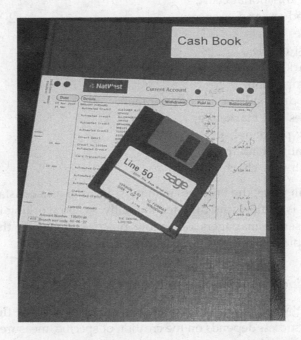

Over recent years the role of dental practice managers has been extended to include financial aspects of practice management in line with managers in other sectors. Previously, practice finances were a closely guarded secret, and the manager's knowledge of the overall financial picture was limited. When permitted to work within income and expenditure targets as set out in the practice business plan, with agreed reporting protocols practice managers can make a meaningful contribution to financial management.

If members of dental teams, with no formal financial management training, are promoted into the role of practice manager, as part of their training they need to develop a working knowledge of financial controls. Their role is not simply to ensure the smooth running of the practice but to maximise practice income and control expenditure so that the practice runs smoothly and profitably meeting the objectives set in the business plan.

The business plan

To quote business guru Sir John Harvey-Jones,

> *'Business is going somewhere, you're either in drive or reverse, there is no park mode.'* A business plan is central if the business is to 'go somewhere'. It must paint a clear picture of the business in words and figures under the following headings:

- business background and direction;
- organisational chart;
- products and services;
- sales targets;
- cost of sales;
- market identification;
- competition;
- product and service development;
- sales and marketing;
- key personnel;
- quality standards;
- cash flow chart.

Once in place, the business plan must be used as a constant point of reference, which is audited and updated annually. When working to an agreed business plan, senior managers can allow practice managers the freedom to define appropriate operational measures for its achievement.

Defining financial management

Since the aim of financial management is to achieve the practice's business goals, success depends on the creation of specific, measured, achievable, agreed, relevant and time-measured targets, based on previous performance, with adjustments built in to reflect financial trends. Financial management begins with the practice vision, expressed as a mission statement in the business plan and broken down into one-, three- and five-year goals, expressed in words and as cash flow forecasts.

The mission statement

The mission statement begins with the practice vision. For example, it may state:

> *'It is the intention of this practice to work with our patients to provide the very best possible standard of both clinical and non-clinical dental care. We aim to provide a friendly, supportive environment in which our patients and colleagues can realise their potential.'*

With a mission statement in place it is possible to plan activities to achieve the vision. The mission statement is therefore a point of reference for decision-making. Funding for activities contributing to the achievement of the vision should be evaluated and considered, whereas those with no obvious impact must be sidelined or discarded.

Cash flow management

The term cash flow refers to the movement of moneys within the business in terms of:

- receipts: moneys received for goods and services;
- payments: moneys paid out to run the business.

In his book, *Finance for the Terrified*, Mike Grace, author, dentist and authority on practice management issues, says,

'A cash flow forecast is a form of budgeting for the business, it provides us with a calculated guess of the income we expect to receive and the costs that we estimate we will have to pay.'

Cash flow management aims to control finances by working within a framework of policies and protocols that define:

- how quickly we pay bills;
- levels of stock held on the premises;
- reconciliation activities;
- performance indicators.

Successfully predicting cash flow activity relies on in-depth knowledge of the business, allowing the manager to predict peaks and troughs.

> At the planning stage, cash flow targets should be broken down into the following three categories:
>
> - short term: plans that come into effect within the next four weeks;
> - middle term: plans that will come into effect over the next six months;
> - long term: plans that will come into effect after six months.

Cash flow forecasts are essential management tools from which management accounts are prepared. The practice owners should view these on a monthly basis so progress can be monitored and future budgets amended in line with known or anticipated variances.

Income

NHS income
For practices working to a Personal Dental Services (PDS) contract, the main source of income will be linked to the contract value negotiated with their

PCT and paid in 12 equal instalments. Practices need to develop fee collection systems because uncollected patient fees represent a loss to the practice. The PCT will provide practices with schedules of patients' charges, which will be deducted from the monthly payments. It is therefore advisable to collect payments from patients before they are treated.

In their publication, *Basic Financial Management for General Dental Practice*, the BDA advises practices that effective income control depends upon the practice maximising its income by:

- presenting patients with an account update at each visit;
- collecting all charges (ask the patient to pay as they receive treatment);
- paying fees collected into the bank account as soon as possible;
- keeping accurate records of running costs.

Private patient income

Non-NHS income will be collected both from the providers of dental schemes (covered in Chapter 9) and directly from patients' private treatment fees. As with NHS fees, accurate records of moneys paid and due must be kept. Practice policy should state when and how patients are to be notified of payments due.

Expenditure

> Expenditure is the money spent to operate the practice. For management and accountancy purposes this is divided into capital and revenue expenditure.
>
> - *Capital expenditure* is the money spent on items with a realisable value (those items that we liquidate (sell and use the funds for the business)).
> - *Revenue expenditure* is the money spent to run the business, e.g. the cost of stock, wages, heating and telephone costs.

Expenditure must be carefully monitored to ensure all purchases are best value for money. It is possible to save money by shopping around suppliers and striking deals. Purchases need to be planned and stock monitored and controlled.

To provide patients with the best possible standard of care, we must meet our team's reasonable financial needs. Wages represent the greatest single practice expense, so care is needed to realise the best possible value from this expenditure. People must have a clear job description setting out what is expected from them in exchange for their salary.

Cashbook

The Inland Revenue requires all businesses to keep a cashbook showing all income and expenditure. The cashbook should be updated daily to provide up to the minute information on income and expenditure. It will show cheques you have issued that have not yet been presented to the drawer's bank, and moneys that you have banked but have not yet appeared on your bank statement. By entering suppliers' invoices in the cashbook you know how much you owe to suppliers, and from the dental patient management software you can calculate how much the practice is owed by patients. By adding this to the cashbook, you complete the overall financial situation. The cashbook can be a part of a computerised accounting package. However, most bookkeepers keep a paper cashbook in addition to their computerised records.

Financial systems

Effective financial management is dependent upon managers creating clear and well communicated systems. These systems and related activities should be written in the practice operations manual and those staff responsible for carrying out procedures should be trained and competent to perform tasks. The systems required for financial management are shown in Table 12.2.

Although dental practices provide health care rather than a clearly defined product, like any other business their financial objective is to provide a high quality service at a profit.

Table 12.2 Systems required for financial management.

Income	Activities
Patient payments	Patient estimates produced Patients asked to pay for treatment at each visit Computerised payment records Receipting payments Bank paying-in protocols Card Payment System (PDQ)
NHS PDS	Budget paid to practice bank account monthly Payments reconciled
Payments from finance companies	Reconciled with claims made Recorded in the accounts package and on the patient's records
Dental scheme payments	Reconciled with claims made, discrepancies followed up
Sale of dental products	Ordering system Stock reconciliation Pricing policy
Appointment book	Failed appointment fees for missed appointments Fees for private patients cancelling with short notice Waiting list for cancellations
Revenue expenditure	

General Bibliography

Armstrong M (2004) *How to Be an Even Better Manager*. Kogan Page, London.

Bandler R and Grindler J (1990) *Frogs into Princes. Neuro-linguistic Programming*. Eden Grove Editions, London.

BDA (2002) *BDA Compendium*, April. BDA, London.

Belbin RM (1993) *Team Roles at Work*. Butterworth Heinemann, London.

Blanchard K (2000) *The One-Minute Manager Meets the Monkey*. Fontana, London.

Covey SR (1989) *The Seven Habits of Successful People*. Simon & Schuster, London.

Crowe SA (1999) *Since Strangling isn't an Option, Dealing with Difficult People*. Perigee, New York.

Decker B (1989) *How to Communicate Effectively*. Kogan Page, London.

Deming WE (1968) *Out of Crisis*. MIT Centre of Advanced Engineering Study, Boston, Mass.

Drucker P (1955) *The Practice of Management: Concepts, Decisions, Cases*. Irwin, New York.

Drucker PF (1993) *The Post-capitalist Society*. Harper Business, New York.

Goleman D (2000) *Working with Emotional Intelligence*. Bloomsbury Press, London.

Handy C (1994) *The Empty Raincoat*. Hutchinson, London.

Honey P and Mumford A (1986) *The Manual of Learning Styles*. Peter Honey, Maidenhead.

James J (2001) *Body Talk at Work*. Piatkus, London.

Kay L and Tinsley S (1996) *Frightening Patients? Frightening Dentists?: Communication for the Dental Team*. Partners in Practice, Brackley.

Lloyd SR (1988) *How to Develop Assertiveness*. Kogan Page, London.

Maslow A (1954) *Motivation and Personality*. Harper & Row, New York.

Newsome P (2001) *The Patient-centred Dental Practice*. BDJ Books, London.

O'Connor J and Seymour J (1993) *Introducing Neuro-Linguisitc Programming*. Thorsons, London.

Rattan R (1996) *Making Sense of Dental Practice Management*. Radcliffe Medical Press, Oxford.

Righton C (2006) *The Life Audit. Take Control of Your Life Now*. Hodder Mobius, London.

Websites

URL	Description
www.Acas.org.uk	Employment information
www.badn.org.uk	British Association of Dental Nurses
www.badt.org.uk	British Association of Dental Therapists
www.bda.org	British Dental Association
www.bdha.org.uk	British Dental Hygienists' Assocation
www.bdpma.org.uk	British Dental Practice Managers Association
www.bdra.org.uk	British Dental Receptionists' Association
www.bdta.org.uk	British Dental Trades Association
www.cdc.gov	Guidelines for infection control in dental health care settings
www.cppih.org	Patient and Public Involvement Forum
www.Dentalhealth.org.uk	British Dental Health Foundation
www.Dentalhelpline.org	Word of Mouth Helpline
www.dh.gov.uk	Department of Health
www.dpb.nhs.uk	Dental Practice Board
www.gdc-uk.org	General Dental Council
www.Hse.gov.uk	Health and safety information
www.nasda.org.uk	British Association of Specialist Dental Accountants
www.nhs.uk	National Health Service
www.nhsdirect.nhs.uk	NHS Direct
www.pals.nhs.uk	Patient Advice and Liaison Service
www.Peoplemanagement.co.uk	General personnel management information

Index